Moving Forward in Critical Care Nursing: Lessons Learned from the COVID-19 Pandemic

Editors

SHARON C. O'DONOGHUE
JUSTIN H. DILIBERO

CRITICAL CARE NURSING CLINICS OF NORTH AMERICA

www.ccnursing.theclinics.com

September 2024 • Volume 36 • Number 3

ELSEVIER

1600 John F. Kennedy Boulevard • Suite 1800 • Philadelphia, Pennsylvania, 19103-2899

http://www.theclinics.com

CRITICAL CARE NURSING CLINICS OF NORTH AMERICA Volume 36, Number 3
September 2024 ISSN 0899-5885, ISBN-13: 978-0-443-12881-3

Editor: Kerry Holland
Developmental Editor: Sukirti Singh

Critical Care Nursing Clinics of North America (ISSN 0899-5885) is published quarterly by Elsevier Inc., 360 Park Avenue South, New York, NY 10010-1710. Months of issue are March, June, September, and December. Business and Editorial Offices: 1600 John F. Kennedy Blvd., Suite 1800, Philadelphia, PA 19103-2899. Periodicals postage paid at New York, NY and additional mailing offices. Subscription prices are $166.00 per year for US individuals, $100.00 per year for US students and residents, $206.00 per year for Canadian individuals, $230.00 per year for international individuals, $115.00 per year for international students/residents and $100.00 per year for Canadian students/residents. For institutional access pricing please contact Customer Service via the contact information below. To receive student/resident rate, orders must be accompanied by name of affiliated institution, data of term, and the *signature* of program/residency coordinator on institution letterhead. Orders will be billed at individual rate until proof of status is received. Foreign air speed delivery is included in all *Clinics* subscription prices. All prices are subject to change without notice. Orders, claims, and journal inquiries: Please visit our Support Hub page https://service.elsevier.com for assistance.

Reprints. For copies of 100 or more of articles in this publication, please contact the Commercial Reprints Department, Elsevier Inc., 360 Park Avenue South, New York, New York, 10010-1710; Tel.: 212-633-3874, Fax: 212-633-3820, and E-mail: reprints@elsevier.com.

Critical Care Nursing Clinics of North America is covered in *MEDLINE/PubMed (Index Medicus), International Nursing Index, Nursing Citation Index, Cumulative Index to Nursing and Allied Health Literature,* and *RNdex Top 100.*

Contributors

EDITORS

SHARON C. O'DONOGHUE, DNP, RN
Nurse Specialist, Professional Development Coordinator, Lois E. Silverman Department of Nursing, Beth Israel Deaconess Medical Center, Boston, Massachusetts, USA

JUSTIN H. DILIBERO, DNP, APRN, CCRN, ACCNS-AG, FCNS
Interim Dean, Zvart Onanian School of Nursing, Rhode Island College, Providence, Rhode Island, USA

AUTHORS

MARIAN ALTMAN, PhD, RN, CNS-BC, CCRN
Nurse Educator, American Association of Critical-Care Nurses, Aliso Viejo, California, USA

JENNIFER BARSAMIAN, DNP, RN, NPD-C
Director, Department of Nursing Clinical and Professional Development, Mount Auburn Hospital, Cambridge, Massachusetts, USA

LEANNE M. BOEHM, PhD, RN, ACNS-BC
Assistant Professor, School of Nursing, Critical Illness, Brain Dysfunction, and Survivorship (CIBS) Center, Vanderbilt University Medical Center, Nashville, Tennessee, USA

KERRY CARNEVALE, DNP, RN
Nurse Specialist for Quality and Safety, Beth Israel Deaconess Medical Center, Boston, Massachusetts, USA

LISA CONNELLY, DNP, RN
Assistant Professor, Zvart Onanian School of Nursing, Rhode Island College, Fogarty Life Science, Providence, Rhode Island, USA

CASEY CUNHA, DNP, RN, CNP
Assistant Professor, Zvart Onanian School of Nursing, Rhode Island College, Fogarty Life Science, Providence, Rhode Island, USA

TENZIN DECHEN, MPH
Biostatistician, Center for Healthcare Delivery Science, Beth Israel Deaconess Medical Center, Boston, Massachusetts, USA

JUSTIN H. DILIBERO, DNP, APRN, CCRN, ACCNS-AG, FCNS
Interim Dean, Zvart Onanian School of Nursing, Rhode Island College, Providence, Rhode Island, USA

KELLY GALLAGHER, MSN, RN, NPD-BC, NEA-BC
Director, Nursing Programs, Nurse Residency Program, Vizient, Inc., Chicago, Illinois, USA

DANIELLE GOTT, MSN, RN
Nurse Specialist, Professional Development, Beth Israel Deaconess Medical Center, Boston, Massachusetts, USA

M. DAVE HANSON†, MSN, RN, ACNS-BC, NEA-BC
Director of Program Strategy and Partnerships, Society of Critical Care Medicine, Chicago, Illinois, USA

SUSAN M. HOLLAND, EdD, MSN, RN, NEA-BC
Nursing Director, Beth Israel Deaconess Medical Center, Boston, Massachusetts, USA

ANNMARIE HOSIE, PhD, RN
Associate Professor, School of Nursing & Midwifery Sydney, University of Notre Dame Australia, Cunningham Centre for Palliative Care, St Vincent's Health Network Sydney, IMPACCT- Improving Palliative, Aged and Chronic Care Through Research and Translation, University of Technology Sydney, Sydney, New South Wales, Australia

TIFFANY KELLEY, PhD, MBA, RN, NI-BC, FNAP
Visiting Associate Professor, Director, Healthcare Innovation Online Graduate Certificate Program, Co-Director, Nursing and Engineering Innovation Center, Affiliate Faculty, Connecticut Center for Entrepreneurship and Innovation, University of Connecticut School of Nursing, Storrs, Connecticut, USA; Founder and CEO, iCare Nursing Solutions and Nightingale Apps, Boston, Massachusetts, USA

SUSAN LACEY, PhD, RN, CNL, FAAN
Associate Director, Society of Critical Care Medicine, Rolling Meadows, Illinois, USA

KATHLEEN M. LUCKNER, MSN, APRN, ACCNS-AG, CCRN
Critical Care Clinical Nurse Specialist, ChristianaCare, Newark, Delaware, USA

KERRI MAYA, PhD(c), MSL, RN, NPD-BC
Director of Continuing Professional Development, Sutter Health System, Sacramento, California, USA

ALLISON MCHUGH, DNP, MHCDS, MS, RN, NE-BC
Assistant Professor and Executive Health Systems Leadership Coordinator, Florida State University, Tallahassee, Florida, USA

CHARLENE MILLER, BSN, RN, CCRN
Nurse Shift Manager; Mercy Medical Center, Redding, California, USA

ASHLEY L. O'DONOGHUE, PhD
Economist, Center for Healthcare Delivery Science, Beth Israel Deaconess Medical Center, Boston, Massachusetts, USA

SHARON C. O'DONOGHUE, DNP, RN
Nurse Specialist, Professional Development Coordinator, Lois E. Silverman Department of Nursing, Beth Israel Deaconess Medical Center, Boston, Massachusetts, USA

AMANDA STEFANCYK OBERLIES, PhD, MBA, RN, FAAN
Chief Executive Officer, Organization of Nurse Leaders MA, RI, CT, NH, VT, Whitinsville, Massachusetts, USA

KATHERINE ORSILLO, MSN, RN
Nurse Specialist, Professional Development, Beth Israel Deaconess Medical Center, Boston, Massachusetts, USA

KELLY M. POTTER, PhD, RN, CNE
Research Assistant Professor, Department of Critical Care Medicine, CRISMA Center, University of Pittsburgh, Pittsburgh, Pennsylvania, USA

BRENDA T. PUN, DNP, RN
Director of Data Quality, Department of Medicine, Pulmonary and Critical Care, Critical Illness, Brain Dysfunction, and Survivorship Center, Vanderbilt University Medical Center, Nashville, Tennessee, USA

ANGELA RENKEMA, MPH, BSN, RN, NPD-BC, CV-BC, CPH
Director, Programmatic Advisory Services (Former), Nurse Residency Program, Vizient, Inc., Chicago, Illinois, USA

MARC SCHIFFMAN, MD
Executive Co-Director, Vascular and Interventional Radiology, Weill Cornell Medicine, New York, New York, USA

MAUREEN A. SECKEL, MSN, APRN, ACNS-BC, CCNS, CCRN, FCCM, FCNS, FAAN
Critical Care Clinical Nurse Specialist and Sepsis Consultant, Christiana Care, Newark, Delaware, USA

CHRISTINE STEWART, MSN, RN, PHN, CCRN-K, CHTP/I
Cardiac Surgery Clinic Manager, Mercy Medical Center, Redding, California, USA

AMBERLY TICOTSKY, MPH, BSN, RN
Nurse Coordinator, Critical Illness and COVID-19 Survivorship Program, Beth Israel Deaconess Medical Center, Boston, Massachusetts, USA

ASHLEY WADDELL, PhD, RN, FAAN
Director, Government Affairs and Educational Programs, Organization of Nurse Leaders MA, RI, CT, NH, VT, Whitinsville, Massachusetts, USA

KAREN WHOLEY, MSN, RN
Assistant Professor, Zvart Onanian School of Nursing, Rhode Island College, Fogarty Life Science, Providence, Rhode Island, USA

STACEY WILLIAMS, DNP, APRN, CPNP-AC
Nurse Practitioner, Pediatric Critical Care Unit, Monroe Carrell Jr Children's Hospital at Vanderbilt, Nashville, Tennessee, USA

BETHANY YOUNG, PhD(c), RN, AGCNS-BC, CCRN
Clinical Nurse Specialist, Department of Nursing, Hospital of the University of Pennsylvania, Philadelphia, Pennsylvania, USA

Contents

Coronavirus disease 2019 (COVID-19) was first identified in December 2019 and quickly became a global pandemic. The understanding of the pathophysiology, treatment, and management of the disease has evolved since the beginning of the pandemic in 2020. COVID-19 can be complicated by immune system dysfunction, lung injury with hypoxemia, acute kidney injury, and coagulopathy. The treatment and management of COVID-19 is based on the severity of illness, ranging from asymptomatic to severe and often life-threatening disease. The 3 main recommended medication classes include antivirals, immunomodulators, and anticoagulants. Other supportive therapies include ensuring adequate oxygenation, mechanical ventilation, and prone positioning.

When exploring the realm of Patient Safety in the context of a COVID-19 global pandemic, the traditional methods of assessment may not be sufficient. This was a crisis that could not be isolated to intensive care units or the hospital environment. In addition to patient safety, one must consider the safety of health care providers and others. Understanding human behavior when faced with a novel disease such as COVID-19 may help prepare for the future when society may once again face a public health crisis together.

Newly licensed registered nurses (NLRNs) were significantly impacted by the COVID-19 pandemic. NLRNs experienced interruptions or significant alterations across, academia, clinical rotations, precepted experiences, and transition to practice programs. All NLRNs were impacted, especially those in critical care who cared for the most acutely ill patients. This article represents a program evaluation of NLRNs in the critical care area during the COVID-19 pandemic and a comprehensive review of the literature related to COVID-19s impact on NLRNs.

The nursing profession has witnessed its share of challenging and trying times including toxic or unhealthy work environments, unsustainable workloads, an aging workforce, inadequate staffing, nurse burnout, staff retention, inadequately trained staff, an increase in workplace violence, and several pandemics. Both individually and collectively, these thorny issues have placed a heavy burden on nurses. Unfortunately, many capable and competent nurses have left the profession altogether, which further compounds an already problematic situation. This article highlights several important strategies for recruiting, retaining, and supporting a high functioning nursing workforce in challenging and trying times.

This article explores current evidence and practical strategies for nurse leaders to advance a healthy work environment. American Association of Critical Care Nurses's Standards for Establishing and Sustaining Healthy Work Environments should guide efforts to reconnect clinical teams with meaningful and satisfying work. Authors propose adding the domain of Wellbeing to guide leaders in holistically addressing the health of all care team members and the work environment.

Clinical nurse educators (CNEs) are expert clinical nurses tasked with supporting the orientation and professional development of nurses on clinical units, yet CNEs themselves often do not receive a formal orientation to support their role transition. CNEs at a large academic medical center participate in a quality improvement program aimed at developing communication skills for difficult conversations, feedback, and debriefing. Findings highlight some of the interpersonal communication challenges CNEs encounter, which endorse the need for a formal CNE orientation and mentoring program.

Nursing documentation is essential to communicate patient care delivery. This review explores available evidence on the contribution of nursing documentation toward quality care delivery during the COVID-19 pandemic. Nine articles were evaluated for at least one of the 6 factors of quality (eg, *safe, timely, equitable, patient-centered, effective, and efficient*). Analysis suggests that right-sizing documentation for optimal care quality requires continued efforts to reinforce the value and need of nursing documentation as a primary data source. Continued practice and research efforts are needed to reframe nursing documentation's essential role in benefiting a patient's current and future health care needs.

Health equity exists when everyone has an equal opportunity to achieve their highest level of health. Effective communication is essential to ensure a therapeutic relationship. Patients with limited English proficiency (LEP) experience communication barriers, leading to poorer outcomes. Federal regulation requires hospitals to provide medically trained interpreters; however, this does not always occur. We identified 3 broad areas of research: communication barriers, outcomes, and costs. Findings highlight the challenges patients with LEP face in the health-care system, and the need for targeted interventions to enhance language access, improve cultural competence among health-care professionals, and ensure equitable outcomes for all.

During the coronavirus disease 2019 pandemic, crisis changes in clinical care increased rates of delirium in the intensive care unit (ICU). Deep sedation, unfamiliar environments with visitor restrictions, and such factors due to high workload and health system strain contributed to the occurrence of delirium doubling in the ICU. As the pandemic wanes, health care systems and ICU leadership must emphasize post-pandemic recovery, integrating lessons learned about delirium management, evidence-based care, and family involvement. Strategies to empower clinicians, creatively deliver care, and integrate families pave the way forward for a more holistic approach to patient care in the post-pandemic era.

Critical care areas saw an unprecedented number of patients throughout the coronavirus disease 2019 (COVID-19) pandemic. Unfortunately, many of these patients continue to experience lingering symptoms long after their discharge from the intensive care unit, related to post-intensive care syndrome and/or post-acute sequelae of COVID-19. Nurses should be aware of these often invisible illnesses and attentive to the fact that this patient population requires ongoing support via multidisciplinary, coordinated care.

This article examines the multifaceted impact of the coronavirus disease 2019 pandemic on nursing education, with a focus on implications for critical care. Issues including the rapid transition to remote learning, stress and burnout, disengagement, challenges in clinical education, ethical dilemmas, and the influence of workforce dynamics on nursing education are discussed. The article explores challenges, opportunities, and the

CRITICAL CARE NURSING CLINICS OF NORTH AMERICA

FORTHCOMING ISSUES

December 2024
Pain Management
Lynn C. Parsons, *Editor*

March 2025
Management of the Hospitalized Patient with Diabetes
Celia Levesque, *Editor*

June 2025
Updates on Human Factors and Technology in the ICU
Shu-Fen Wung, *Editor*

RECENT ISSUES

June 2024
Neonatal Nursing: Clinical Concepts and Practice Implications, Part 2
Leslie Altimier, *Editor*

March 2024
Neonatal Nursing: Clinical Concepts and Practice Implications, Part 1
Leslie Altimier, *Editor*

December 2023
Older Adults in Critical Care
Deborah Garbee, *Editor*

SERIES OF RELATED INTEREST

Nursing Clinics of North America http://www.nursing.theclinics.com

Preface

Resilience and Innovation: Reflection on Critical Care Nursing Through the COVID-19 Era

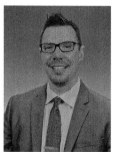

Justin H. DiLibero, DNP, APRN, CCRN, ACCNS-AG, FCNS   Sharon C. O'Donoghue, DNP, RN

Editors

This issue of the *Critical Care Nursing Clinics of North America* is dedicated to the critical care community, who led us through the unprecedented challenges of the COVID-19 pandemic. The pandemic has profoundly impacted individuals, families, the broader health care environment, and especially, the acute and critical care community.

During the initial period, we faced issues of uncertainty related to the disease process, treatment strategies, and infection control measures. We faced the need to rapidly implement evidence-based practices that evolved seemingly by the minute, while stretching resources to meet surging volumes of critically ill patients. The critical care community responded to the emergence of the pandemic, displaying extraordinary resilience, innovation, and adaptability. As the pandemic extended into the following months and years, the critical care community met the extended challenges and changing dynamics with an equally unwavering moral courage, and uncompromising commitment to patient safety.

This issue of *Critical Care Nursing Clinics of North America* serves as a collection of knowledge, insights, and experiences of critical care nursing leaders across the areas of practice, education, and research. These authors have graciously shared their knowledge and insight to improve our understanding of the unique challenges and innovative solutions. This issue covers a comprehensive range of topics, such as quality and safety, implementation science, clinical documentation practice, emergency preparedness, changing demographics, the nursing shortage, systems challenges, and implications for practice, education, and leadership. Each article provides up-

Crit Care Nurs Clin N Am 36 (2024) xiii–xiv
https://doi.org/10.1016/j.cnc.2024.01.001
0899-5885/24/© 2024 Published by Elsevier Inc.

to-date information and evidence-based practices intended to provide new insight and support the highest quality of care as we emerge in the postpandemic era.

Undoubtedly, the pandemic has taken a tremendous toll on individuals, families, and communities; however, amidst adversity, we have also witnessed unparalleled displays of compassion, community, and solidarity. This issue is a testament to those who stand at the forefront, providing life-saving care and comfort to acute and critically ill patients and their families. It is our hope that the articles within provide the opportunity for reflection and healing, deepen our understanding of COVID-19, foster a spirit of collaboration, and inspire innovation toward the advancement of critical care nursing practice, leadership, and education.

With heartfelt appreciation and respect for the acute and critical care nursing community,

Justin H. DiLibero, DNP, APRN, CCRN, ACCNS-AG, FCNS
Rhode Island College
Onanian School of Nursing
600 Mount Pleasant Avenue, Office 158
Providence, RI 02908, USA

Sharon C. O'Donoghue, DNP, RN
Lois E. Silverman Department of Nursing
Beth Israel Deaconess Medical Center
330 Brookline Avenue
Boston, MA 02215, USA

E-mail addresses:
jdilibero@ric.edu (J.H. DiLibero)
shacmol@gmail.com (S.C. O'Donoghue)

Understanding the Evolving Pathophysiology of Coronavirus Disease 2019 and Adult Nursing Management

Kathleen M. Luckner, MSN, APRN, ACCNS-AG, CCRN[a,1,*],
Maureen A. Seckel, MSN, APRN, ACNS-BC, CCNS, CCRN, FCCM, FCNS, FAAN[b]

KEYWORDS

- COVID-19 • Coronavirus • SARS-CoV-2 • Evidenced-based practice
- Pathophysiology

KEY POINTS

This article provides a review of the evidence related to the

- History and pathophysiology of severe acute respiratory syndrome coronavirus 2 (SARS-CoV-2).
- Medication management in patients with coronavirus disease 2019 (COVID-19), and
- Latest research related to the care of adult COVID-19 patients.

INTRODUCTION

Coronavirus disease 2019 (COVID-19) was first discovered in China in December 2019 and by March 2020 it was identified as a pandemic by the World Health Organization. Manifestation of COVID-19 illness ranges from asymptomatic carriers to critical illness progressing to multiorgan failure and death.[1] COVID-19 is caused by the ribonucleic acid (RNA) virus severe acute respiratory syndrome coronavirus 2 (SARS-CoV-2), which is predominantly spread from person-to-person through respiratory secretions and droplets produced through coughing, sneezing, or talking. Spread is worse in areas with inadequate ventilation as aerosols can remain for hours and can travel to surfaces, where the virus can live for up to 6 days.[2] Viral entry into the body is through the upper respiratory tract and lung pneumocytes, leading to primary viral replication. Viremia disseminates the virus to other organs which results in a secondary replication. COVID-19

[a] ChristianaCare, 4755 Ogletown-Stanton Road, Newark, DE 19713, USA; [b] MSeckel Consultant, 2 Fox Lane, Newark, DE 19711, USA
[1] Present address: 400 Foulk Road Apartment 4A9, Wilmington, DE 19803, USA
* Corresponding author.
E-mail address: Kathleen.m.luckner@christianacare.org

Crit Care Nurs Clin N Am 36 (2024) 295–321
https://doi.org/10.1016/j.cnc.2024.01.002
0899-5885/24/© 2024 Elsevier Inc. All rights reserved.
ccnursing.theclinics.com

infection typically presents with symptoms of fever, cough, sore throat, fatigue, and malaise. More severe cases can result in dyspnea related to pneumonitis, hypoxemia, and respiratory failure. Risk factors for poorer outcomes include advanced age, obesity, diabetes, hypertension, cardiovascular disease, smoking, cancer, and autoimmune diseases.[2,3]

PATHOPHYSIOLOGY

SARS-CoV-2 is a single-stranded RNA virus. It enters host cells through cytoprotease transmembrane protease serine 2 (TM-PRSS2), a factor required for cell entry, and through angiotensin-converting enzyme 2(ACE2) receptors, using a spike (S) glycoprotein for attachment.[1,2,4] ACE2 receptors are mainly found in type II alveolar cells, bronchial epithelial cells, myocardial cells, renal tubules, liver cholangiocytes, neurons, and many other sites.[5] SARS-CoV-2 attacks several organs expressing ACE2 receptors, including the heart, brain, blood vessels, liver, kidney, and, most significantly, the lungs.[6] After binding to ACE2 receptors, TMPRSS2 proteases cleave the spike protein of the virus, which allows viral entry and replication.[4]

SARS-CoV-2 survives and replicates inside macrophages.[7] Compared to DNA viruses, RNA viruses are commonly more susceptible to mutation; therefore, SARS-CoV-2 is constantly evolving and mutating. The future of COVID-19 is dependent upon the virological diversity, spread, and clinical characteristics of these variants.[2]

Cytokine Storm

SARS-CoV-2 infection triggers the body's natural immune response. The adaptive immune system manages the infection through B-cells, which produce antibodies, CD4+ T cells, which aid in viral clearance, and CD8+ T cells, which defend through a variety of cytokines.[4]

Cytokines are polypeptides that are essential for the correct functioning of the immune system and are involved in processes such as inflammation, tissue repair, fibrosis, and coagulation. However, immune system dysfunction can cause an acute overproduction and uncontrolled release of pro-inflammatory markers, both locally and systemically, called a cytokine storm.[6–8] Activated macrophages can produce various proinflammatory cytokines such as tumor necrosis factor (TNF) α, interleukin (IL)-1, IL-6, IL-17, and IL-18. These cytokines may trigger the inflammatory cascade, generating a cytokine storm.[7,8]

Manifestations of cytokine storm vary but include high fever, fatigue, headache, arthralgia, and diarrhea. It can evolve to impaired coagulation, acute respiratory distress syndrome (ARDS), acute kidney injury (AKI), and liver damage.[7] Cytokine storm is associated with microvascular and macrovascular complications related to endothelial dysfunction, including myocardial infarction and stroke.[4]

Severe COVID-19 is associated with elevated cytokine levels, specifically IL-1β, IL-6, IL-2R, and TNF-α.[4,9] Elevated IL-6 cytokine levels can lead to multiorgan failure and are associated with increased intensive care unit (ICU) admission, ARDS, and mortality.[4,8]

COVID-19 causes the production of autoantibodies against several immune-modulatory proteins. Therefore, in the earlier phase of COVID-19 infection, the immune system might not be able to efficiently clear infected cells and could even favor the replication of the virus. In a later phase of infection, the immune system recovers the ability to effectively fight the virus.[7] However, because the virus has been able to replicate, the immune system would produce an exaggerated reaction.[7]

SARS-CoV-2 infection of lung cells, in particular type II pneumocytes, can cause inflammatory cell infiltrate, consisting of neutrophils, macrophages, CD8+ and CD4+ T lymphocytes, and mass production of cytokines. This process often leads to pneumonia, ARDS, and multiorgan damage.[4,7,9] Because of this, management of cytokine release and prevention of subsequent infections may be a beneficial approach for COVID-19 therapy.

Coronavirus Disease 2019 Lung Injury

Lung injury from COVID-19 may result from direct viral damage and thrombotic and inflammatory reactions related to host defense response.[3] This lung damage can result in pulmonary edema, diffuse alveolar injury, presence of reactive type II pneumocyte hyperplasia, fibrinous exudates, monocytes/macrophages within the alveolar spaces, and inflammatory infiltration of interstitial mononuclear cells.[9] Excessive local release of cytokines leads to epithelial and endothelial cell damage and is the determinant of pathologic alterations and clinical manifestations of ARDS.[3,9] About 15% to 30% of COVID-19 patients progress to severe ARDS within 8 days of initial symptoms.[9,10]

The SARS-CoV-2 virus attaches to ACE2 in the alveolar epithelium and vascular endothelium resulting in interstitial edema and alveolar fluid filling. Smokers and the elderly tend to have a higher number of ACE2 receptors, and therefore are more susceptible to COVID-19 infection and subsequent ARDS.[11] COVID-19 lung damage related to ARDS can result in diffuse alveolar damage, interstitial edema, alveolar hemorrhage, endothelial cell injury, and reduced lung parenchymal compliance. Greater vasculopathy, including macrothrombosis and microthrombosis, has been seen in COVID-19.[3] Autopsy of patients with severe SARS-CoV-2 infection reveals the presence of diffuse alveolar damage with a higher thrombus burden in pulmonary capillaries.[12]

COVID-19 imaging reveals peripheral and basilar ground-glass opacities in early disease, progressing to typical consolidation as in ARDS.[3,10] This disease process results in better lung compliance in early COVID-19 lung injury. Surfactant-producing alveolar epithelial type II cells express ACE-2. With injury and release of these stores, the compliance declines with microvascular leakage.[3]

Hypoxemia, Hypercapnia, and Dyspnea in Coronavirus Disease 2019 Lung Injury

Hypoxemia in COVID-19 is caused by low ventilation to perfusion (V/Q) mismatch and shunt. The V/Q mismatch contributes to rising carbon dioxide (CO2) dead space. In COVID-19 lung injury, reported values of dead space are as high as 75%, largely due to vascular obstruction.[3,13]

Silent hypoxemia, sometimes referred to as happy hypoxia, is commonly seen in COVID-19. Silent hypoxemia denotes arterial hypoxemia in patients with a lack of dyspnea and can occur for a few reasons. Fever, which is a common symptom of COVID-19, causes a left shift in the oxygen dissociation curve leading to a lower SaO2 with any given Pao_2 (**Fig. 1**). This shift causes desaturations without a change in chemoreceptor stimulation, resulting in silent hypoxemia.[14] In addition, many COVID-19 patients are elderly and have diabetes. Both of these factors can result in a diminished signaling from peripheral and central chemoreceptors in response to arterial Pco_2 and Po_2 changes.[3,14] Silent hypoxemia can be a significant threat for patients who are told to seek care if they are dyspneic. Prolonged unrecognized hypoxemia can lead to deterioration and death.

Coronavirus Disease 2019 and Acute Kidney Injury

While COVID-19 typically causes hypoxemia and respiratory failure, renal involvement occurs in about 30% of hospitalized COVID-19 patients and is the most common extrapulmonary complication.[15] COVID-19 not only causes new kidney disease but can complicate treatment and increase mortality rates in people with existing kidney

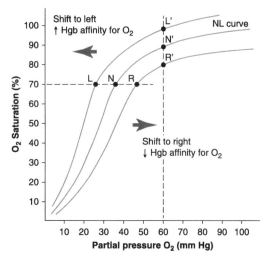

Fig. 1. Oxyhemoglobin dissociation curve. A Pao$_2$ of 60 mmHg correlates with an oxygen saturation of 90%. When the Pao$_2$ falls below 60 mmHg, small changes in Pao$_2$ are reflected in large changes in oxygen saturation. Shifts in oxyhemoglobin curve are shown. L, left shift; N, normal; Pao$_2$, partial pressure of oxygen; R, right shift. (*From* Alspach J. AACN Instructor's Resource Manual for AACN Core Curriculum for Critical Care Nursing. 5th ed. Philadelphia: Saunders; 2001).

disease.[4] The majority of COVID-19 patients with AKI have acute tubular necrosis, although some patients also have acute interstitial nephritis, microthrombi in the kidney vessels, and focal segmental glomerulosclerosis.[15]

The 3 main pathophysiological causes of AKI in COVID-19 patients are hemodynamic abnormalities, hypoxia, and cytokine storm.[4] SARS-CoV-2 has an increased affinity for the receptor protein ACE2. The ACE2 receptor protein is found throughout the body and is highly expressed in the proximal kidney tubules. SARS-CoV-2's increased affinity for the ACE2 receptor protein could cause kidney injury. Minor injury to the tubules can be worsened by hemodynamic instability.

Cytokine release, in response to COVID-19, affects local inflammatory response, pathogen clearance, and thrombosis which lead to microcirculatory and endothelial dysfunction and increased renal interstitial pressure. This increased pressure can cause damage to the tubules and acute tubular necrosis.[4,7] Additionally, IL-6, TNF-α, and Fas ligand are inflammatory mediators that directly cause harm to renal and tubule endothelial cells by binding to their receptors.[4]

Coronavirus Disease 2019 and Coagulopathy

Increased rates of thrombotic complications, including microvascular thrombosis, venous thromboembolism (VTE), and arterial thrombus are associated with COVID-19.[1] Coagulopathy associated with COVID-19 has been shown to correlate with disease severity and increased mortality.[1]

Intact endothelium plays an important role in maintaining hemostasis; however, SARS-CoV-2 infection results in endothelial damage. Direct viral infection with SARS-CoV-2 can lead to diffuse endothelial inflammation, apoptosis, and pyroptosis.[1,16,17] Endothelium can also be damaged by cytokines, hypoxia, and complement activation. These result in the activation of coagulation system through exposure of thrombogenic basement membrane, release of factor VIII, von Willebrand factor, and activated platelets.[1] Endothelium dysfunction leads to coagulopathy. Markers of endothelial cell activation have been significantly higher in ICU patients with severe COVID-19 compared to non-ICU patients.[1]

As part of the immune defense, neutrophils release neutrophil extracellular traps (NETs). NETs amplify platelet activation and aggregation and cause thrombin activation. In lung tissue, NETs are associated with microthrombi and platelet deposition.[1,16] This suggests that NETs play an important role in coagulopathy/thrombosis associated with COVID-19.

The complement system is a key mediator of the immune response. Anaphylatoxins recruit and activate neutrophils, monocytes, endothelial cells, and platelets. This results in the release of proinflammatory cytokines, which promote coagulation. The complement system, by leading to widespread microvascular thrombosis, could play a role in the coagulopathy associated with COVID-19.[1,16]

COVID-19 is associated with a high incidence of venous and arterial thrombotic complications. While VTE accounts for the majority of these events, stroke and acute myocardial infarction also occur. The occurrence of VTE in critically ill COVID-19 patients is high and is closely related to disease severity and clinical prognosis.[16] The prevalence of pulmonary embolism is disproportionately high compared to deep VTE. This suggests primary in-situ pulmonary thrombus, rather than an embolism.[1] In severe COVID-19 disease, virus proliferation within the lung tissue can contribute to the in situ activation of lung megakaryocyte–derived platelets. Platelet activation and ensuring microthrombus formation in the lung vasculature further aggravate pulmonary inflammation.[17]

EVIDENCED-BASED MANAGEMENT
Classification

Adult COVID-19 outpatients and inpatients are classified using clinical symptoms to align severity with treatment recommendations in multiple guidelines[18–21] (**Table 1**).

Table 1
Severity of illness in coronavirus disease 2019 patients

Category	Clinical Indicators
Asymptomatic or Presymptomatic	Positive test but have no symptoms
Mild	Signs and symptoms such as fever, cough, sore throat, malaise, headache, muscle pain, nausea, vomiting, diarrhea, and loss of taste and smell but *do not have shortness of breath, dyspnea, or abnormal chest x ray*
Moderate	Evidence of lower respiratory disease (clinical assessment or imaging) and who have SpO2 $\geq$ 94%[18] or > 94%[20] on room air
Severe	SpO2 < 94%[18], $\leq$ 94%[20], <90%[21] on room air, Pao_2/Fio_2 ratio < 300 mmHg, respiratory rate > 30 breaths/min, pneumonia, lung infiltrates > 50%, signs of respiratory distress
Critical	Respiratory failure, septic shock, and/or multi-organ failure Examples include mechanical ventilation, ECMO, or ARDS

Abbreviations: ARDS, acute respiratory distress syndrome; ECMO, extracorporeal membrane oxygenation; Fio_2, fraction of inspired oxygen; Pao_2, partial pressure of oxygen; SpO2, saturation of peripheral oxygen.
Data from Refs.[18,20,21]

While the classifications are similar, there are subtle differences in the severity of illness definitions between guidelines. A recent meta-analysis of randomized controlled trials recommended standardizing definitions across research and management in order to maximize our understanding of outcomes.[22] Along with clinical symptoms, oxygenation or degree of hypoxemia is central to defining severity in COVID-19.

Emergency Use Authorization

Therapy has evolved from the start of the pandemic in 2019 to current-day recommendations based on research. Many therapeutics were initially implemented under the US Food and Drug Administration (FDA) Emergency Use Authorization (EUA) due to the rapid spread and severity of the pandemic, with some now having full FDA approval, others having approval under revised EUAs, and others being no longer recommended. Drugs or devices that are under EUA are first recommended by the US Department of Health and Human Services Secretary for public health emergency use and then evaluated by the FDA regarding risks and benefits before issuing an EUA.[23] The prescribing provider for any EUA must complete all mandatory requirements prior to administration including providing a fact sheet to the patient and or caregiver, informed consent that an EUA is an unapproved medication, and the risks and benefits.[23] All medication errors and serious adverse events potentially related to the medication must also be reported. EUA is not the same as FDA approval or licensure and any EUA undergoes ongoing re-evaluation.[24] In May 2023, the COVID-19 status as a public emergency under the Public Health Services (PHS) Act expired. However, the end of the PHS Act does not impact the FDA's ability to continue to authorize treatments for emergency use and evaluate new EUA's when criteria is met.[24] The complete list of all current EUAs is available at https://www.fda.gov/drugs/emergency-preparedness-drugs/emergency-use-authorizations-drugs-and-non-vaccine-biological-products.

Medications

There are 3 major classifications of medications specific to recommended care in COVID-19 patients. These include antivirals, immunomodulators, and anticoagulants. Many other medications may be involved in the care of these patients specific to their underlying disease conditions (**Table-2**).

Antivirals

In general, antiviral drugs work by inhibiting virus replication. There are currently 4 antiviral treatment recommendations. Ritonavir-boosted nirmatrelvir is a combination 3-pill oral medication that should be implemented within 5 days of COVID-19 symptoms in outpatients who have high risk of progressing to severe COVID-19.[25] This combination drug was approved by the FDA in 2023 for adult patients and requires an EUA for pediatric patients.[26] The main component, nirmatrelvir, inhibits protease which is essential in viral replication and has been shown to be effective against all coronaviruses.[18] The second component, ritonavir, is a strong cytochrome P450 3A4 (CYP3A4) inhibitor which is used to boost nirmatrelvir to a targeted therapeutic range. In the EPIC-HR large randomized controlled trial in unvaccinated subjects, results showed that nirmatrelvir with ritonavir had an 89.1% relative risk reduction in hospitalization or death in patients at high risk for progression to severe COVID-19 without significant adverse events.[27] However, due to the known interactions with medications that are metabolized or induced by CYP3A4, there are drug interactions that may lead either to drug toxicities or potential for loss of virologic response.[25] All patient

Table 2
Coronavirus disease 2019 adult medications dosing recommendations

	FDA or EUA	Action and Use	Dose and Route	Contraindications/Warnings	Side Effects	Pregnancy/Lactation
Antivirals						
Remdesivir (Veklury®)	FDA-approved	Administer as soon as possible after diagnosis and meets clinical criteria. Severe acute respiratory distress coronavirus 2 (SARS-CoV-2) nucleotide analog RNA polymerase inhibitor for adults and pediatric patient (28 d of age and at least 3 kg) hospitalized or nonhospitalized with mild to moderate COVID-19 and at risk for progression to severe COVID-19.	Adults Initial, 200 mg IV on day 1 for all patients followed by 100 mg per d, following recommendations. • Nonhospitalized 100 mg IV for total of 3 d. • Hospitalized 100 mg IV for total of 5 d, • Hospitalized with MV or ECMO 100 mg IV for total of 10 d	• History of clinically significant hypersensitivity • Increased risk of transaminase elevation • Risk of reduced antiviral activity when co-administered with chloroquine phosphate or hydroxychloroquine sulfate	Nausea, and ALT and AST increase	Recommended if indicated and should include a discussion of risks and benefits. Lactation can continue.

(continued on next page)

Table 2
(continued)

	FDA or EUA	Action and Use	Dose and Route	Contraindications/Warnings	Side Effects	Pregnancy/Lactation
Ritonavir-boosted nirmatrelvir (Paxlovid®)	FDA-approved for mild to moderate COVID-19 in nonhospitalized adults who are high risk for progression to severe disease including hospitalization and death within 5 d of symptom onset. EUA for treatment of hospitalized adults for a diagnosis other that COVID-19 with mild to moderate COVID-19 and is at high risk for progression to severe disease and within 5 d of symptom onset.	Administer as soon as possible after diagnosis and within 5 d of symptom onset. Combination drug. Nirmatrelvir is an oral protease inhibitor with antiviral activity against all coronaviruses. Ritonavir is a strong cytochrome P450 (CYP- 3A4 inhibitor and pharmacokinetic boosting agent.	300 mg nirmatrelvir (2–150 mg tablets) po and 100 mg ritonavir (1 tablet) po twice daily for 5 d. All 3 tablets should be taken together. May be given with or without food.	• History of clinically significant hypersensitivity to either of components • Dose reduction for moderate renal impairment (eGFR ≥30 to <60 mL/min of 150 mg nirmatrelvir and 100 mg ritonavir • Not recommended in patients with severe renal impairment (eGFR <30 mL/min • Not recommended in patients with severe hepatic impairment (Child-Pugh Class C) • Increased risk of HIV-1 resistance to HIV protease inhibitors in patients with uncontrolled or undiagnosed HIV Ritonavir is a strong CYP3A4 inhibitor and may increase plasma concentrations of medications metabolized by CYP3A. Medications that induce CYP3A may decrease concentration	Dysgeusia Diarrhea, increase in hepatic transaminase, clinical hepatitis, and jaundice	Recommended if indicated and should include a discussion of risks and benefits. Lactation can continue.

| Molnupiravir (Lagevrio®) | EUA for the treatment of mild to moderate COVID-19 in certain adults who are at high risk for progressing to severe COVID-19, including hospitalization and death, and for whom alternative COVID-19 treatment options are not accessible or clinically appropriate. | Administer as soon as possible after diagnosis and within 5 d of symptom onset for patients who are not hospitalized. Nucleoside analog that inhibits SARS-CoV-2 replication for adults only. | 800 mg (4–200 mg capsules) po every 12 h for 5 d.
• With or without food
• May be given via nasogastric or orogastric tube by dissolving capsule content in water | • History of clinically significant hypersensitivity
• Embryo-fetal toxicity
• Bone and cartilage toxicity, not recommended under 18 y of age due to possible effects on bone and cartilage growth | Diarrhea, nausea, and dizziness | Recommended against use in pregnancy. Breastfeeding not recommended during treatment and for 4 d after the last dose. Females of childbearing age should use a reliable method of contraception for duration of treatment and for 4 d after the last dose. Males of reproduction potential should use a reliable method of contraception during treatment and for at least 3 mo after the last dose. |

(continued on next page)

Table 2
(continued)

	FDA or EUA	Action and Use	Dose and Route	Contraindications/Warnings	Side Effects	Pregnancy/Lactation
CCP	EUA for outpatients and hospitalized patients who are immunocompromised. EUA limited to high-titer CCP. Current guidelines state there is insufficient evidence to recommend for or against the use of high-titer CCP in hospitalized or nonhospitalized immunocompromised patients.	Human plasma from recovered COVID-19 patients with high titers of anti–SARS-CoV-2 antibodies.	Administer CCP (~200 mL) through a peripheral or central venous catheter according to institutional practices for plasma administration.	May be contraindicated in patients with history of severe allergic or anaphylaxis to plasma transfusions	Transfusion-transmitted infections (eg, HIV, hepatitis B, hepatitis C), allergic reactions, anaphylaxis, febrile nonhemolytic reactions, TRALI, TACO, hemolytic reactions, hypothermia, metabolic complications, and post-transfusion purpura.	Insufficient data to evaluate risk of major birth defects, miscarriage, or adverse maternal or fetal outcomes Should only be used if the potential benefit outweighs the potential risks. Insufficient data to evaluate whether anti–SARS-CoV-2 antibodies are excreted in milk. Consider risks and benefits.
Immunomodulators						
Dexamethasone	FDA-approved	Anti-inflammatory corticosteroid in hospitalized patients requiring oxygen, NIV, MV, ECMO	6 mg IV or po daily for up to 10 d or until discharge if sooner • Administer po with meals Note: An equivalent dose of an alternative glucocorticoid may be substituted if dexamethasone is unavailable, and dosing is dependent on half-life.	Contraindications include hypersensitivity and/or systemic fungal infections	Adrenal insufficiency, fluid retention, electrolyte disturbances, hypertension, risk of GI perforation. Caution in patients with history ocular herpes simplex due to risk of corneal perforation.	Recommended if indicated.

		• Prednisone 40 mg (daily or 2 divided doses) • Methylprednisolone 32 mg (daily or 2 divided doses) • Hydrocortisone 160 mg (2–4 divided doses daily)			Recommended if indicated and should include a discussion of risks and benefits. Lactation can continue.
Tocilizumab (Actemra®)	Interleukin-6 (IL-6) receptor antagonist	FDA-approved for the treatment of COVID-19 hospitalized adults who are receiving systemic corticosteroids and require supplemental oxygen, NIV, MV, or ECMO.	8 mg/kg IV over 60 min. If clinical signs or symptoms worsen or do not improve after the first dose, 1 additional dose may be given at least 8 h after initial infusion. Doses exceeding 800 mg per infusion are not recommended.	Not recommended in patients with absolute neutrophil count (ANC) below 1000 per mm^3, platelet count below 50,000 per mm^3, or ALT or AST above 10 times the upper limit of normal. Contraindicated in patients with known hypersensitivity. Do not administer during an active infection including localized infection; most patients who developed were taking concomitant immunosuppressants. Use in caution in patients at risk for GI perforation. Monitor for hepatic injury. Avoid use of live vaccines.	Upper respiratory infections, nasopharyngitis, headache, hypertension, increased ALT, and injection site reactions

(continued on next page)

Table 2
(continued)

	FDA or EUA	Action and Use	Dose and Route	Contraindications/ Warnings	Side Effects	Pregnancy/ Lactation
Baricitinib (Olumiant®)	FDA-approved for the treatment of COVID-19 hospitalized patients requiring supplemental oxygen, NIV, MV, or ECMO (5/10/22)	JAK inhibitor indicated for the treatment of hospitalized COVID-19 patients with oxygen, NIV, MV, or ECMO	4 mg po daily up to 14 d or hospital discharge. Tablets may be dispersed in water and given orally, via gastric, nasogastric, or orogastric tube. If tablets are crushed to facilitate dispersion, they should be prepared under ventilated enclosures or PPE. Dosing modifications recommended for renal impairment for moderate and severe renal impairment	Not recommended in patients with absolute lymphocyte count is < 200 cells/ml or absolute neutrophil count (ANC) < 500 cell/ ml. Contraindicated in patients with known hypersensitivity. Should not be given to patients with active tuberculosis. Patients should be screened for viral hepatitis and monitor for hepatic injury. Use in caution in patients at risk for GI perforation. Avoid use with live vaccines. Not recommended for patients with end-stage renal disease, patients on hemodialysis or AKI.	Increase in liver enzymes, thrombocytosis, creatine phosphokinase, and neutropenia DVT, PE, and UTI. Monitor for new infections.	Recommended if indicated and should include a discussion of potential risks and benefits. Lactation should be avoided while taking and for 4 d after the last dose.

Drug	Class	Indication	Dosing	Warnings/Contraindications	Adverse Effects	Pregnancy/Lactation
Vilobelimab (Gohibic®)	Anti-C5a monoclonal antibody	EUA for the treatment of COVID-19 in hospitalized adults when initiated within 48 h of receiving IMV or ECMO. Not available for any other indication. Insufficient evidence to recommend for or against.	800 mg IV over 30–60 min for a maximum of 6 doses. Day 1 is within 48 h of intubation followed by day 2, 4, 8, 15, and 22 as long as patient is still hospitalized.	Associated with an increase of serious infections such as bacterial, fungal, and viral. Contraindicated in patients with known hypersensitivity.	Pneumonia, sepsis, delirium, PE, hypertension, pneumothorax, DVT, herpes simplex, enterococcal infections, UTI, hypoxia, thrombocytopenia, pneumomediastinum, respiratory tract infections, SVT, constipation, and rash	No available data on use in pregnant women Lactation: discontinue drug or nursing, taking into consideration risks and benefits to mother.
Abatacept (Orencia®)	Selective T-cell co-stimulation modulator studied in moderate to severe hospitalized COVID-19 patients.	Off-label use, recommended for hospitalized COVID-19 patients who require conventional oxygen, HFNC, or NIV.	10 mg/kg IV single dose.	Concomitant use with a TNF antagonist can increase the risk of infection. Hypersensitivity reaction. Screen for latent TB and viral hepatitis prior to initiating. Live vaccines should not be given concurrently or within 3 mo of discontinuation.	Headache, upper respiratory tract infection, nasopharyngitis, nausea, anemia, hypertension, CMV reactivation, CMV infection, pyrexia, pneumonia, epistaxis, decreased CD4 lymphocytes, hypermagnesemia, and AKI.	Recommended if indicated and should include a discussion of risks and benefits. Lactation can continue.

(continued on next page)

Table 2
(continued)

	FDA or EUA	Action and Use	Dose and Route	Contraindications/Warnings	Side Effects	Pregnancy/Lactation
Infliximab (Remicade®)	Off-label use, recommended for hospitalized COVID-19 patient who require conventional oxygen, HFNC, or NIV.	Tumor necrosis factor-alpha inhibitor studied for the treatment of hospitalized patients with moderate to severe COVID-19.	5 mg/kg IV single dose.	If an infection develops, monitor carefully and stop if it becomes serious. Screen for hepatitis B prior to therapy. Live vaccines should not be given concurrently. See prescribing information for complete listing.	Infections (upper respiratory, sinusitis, and pharyngitis), infusion-related reactions, headaches, and abdominal pain.	Recommended if indicated and should include a discussion of risks and benefits. Lactation can continue.
Tofacitinib (Xeljanz®)	Off-label use, recommended for hospitalized COVID-19 patients for use in combination with dexamethasone if no other immunomodulatory therapy is available or feasible to use.	JAK inhibitor studies in the treatment of hospitalized COVID-19 patients with pneumonia without NIV, invasive MV, ECMO, or history or current thrombosis.	10 mg po twice daily for up to 14 d or hospital discharge, whichever comes first.	Avoid use in patients with ANC< 500–1000 cells/mm^3, or Hgl<9 g/dL. Requires dose modification when given with strong CYP3A4 inhibitors or moderate CYP34 A inhibitor with strong CYP2C19 Administration with strong CYP3A4 inducers is not recommended	Monitor for new infections.	Unknown in COVID-19

| Sarilumab (Kevzara®) | Off-label use, recommended for hospitalized COVID-19 patients for use in combination with dexamethasone if no other immunomodulatory therapy is available or feasible to use. IV formulation is not approved by the FDA but was used in clinical trials for COVID-19. | Interleukin-6 inhibitor studied in the treatment of hospitalized COVID-19 patients with severe disease. | 400 mg IV over 1 h within 4 h of preparation through central line or peripheral IV. Unknown compatibility and recommended in single IV. | Serious infections have occurred. Monitor laboratory results for neutropenia, thrombocytopenia, liver enzymes, and lipids. GI perforation may be increased with concurrent use of NSAIDs or corticosteroids. Hypersensitivity reactions. Avoid use with live vaccines. | Neutropenia, increased ALT, injection site erythema, upper respiratory infections, UTIs, and leukopenia. | Unknown in COVID-19 |

Abbreviations: AKI, acute kidney injury; ALT, alanine transaminase; ANC, absolute neutrophil count; AST, aspartate transaminase; CCP, COVID-19 convalescent plasma; CD4, clusters of differentiation 4; CMV, cytomegalovirus; COVID-19, coronavirus disease 2019; CYP, cytochrome; DVT, deep vein thrombosis; ECMO, extracorporeal membrane oxygenation; eGFR, estimated glomerular filtration rate; EUA, Emergency Use Authorization; FDA, US Food and Drug Administration; GI, gastrointestinal; HFNC, high-flow nasal cannula; hgl, hemoglobin; HIV, human immunodeficiency virus; IV, intravenous; JAK, janus kinase; kg, kilogram; mg, milligram; mL, milliliter; MV, mechanical ventilation; NIV, noninvasive ventilation; NSAIDs, nonsteroidal anti-inflammatory drugs; PE, pulmonary embolus; PO, orally; PPE, personal protective equipment; RNA; ribonucleic acid; SUBQ, subcutaneous; SVT, supraventricular tachycardia; TACO, transfusion-associated circulatory overload; TB, tuberculosis; TRALI, transfusion-related acute lung injury; UTI, urinary tract infection.

Data from Refs.[18,50,52–55]

medications should be reviewed for potential drug-drug interactions by the provider prior to prescribing and administration.

Another antiviral, remdesivir, works by terminating RNA transcription and is administered by intravenous (IV) infusion within 7 days of symptoms and was the first treatment for COVID-19 approved by the FDA in 2020.[26,28] The duration varies by severity of illness and is 3 days for outpatients, 5 days for most inpatients, and 10 days for severely ill patients needing mechanical ventilation (MV), extracorporeal membrane oxygenation (ECMO), or who have little clinical improvement after the first 5 days of remdesivir.[18] Inpatients should receive a loading dose of 200 mg via IV followed by 100 mg via IV daily for the duration of therapy. An early study in 2020 demonstrated a shortened time to recovery and lower incidence among patients with respiratory tract infection compared to placebo.[29] In a large retrospective cohort study, remdesivir treatment was associated with a statistically significant 17% reduction in inpatient mortality.[30] Due to reports of mild to moderate increases in transaminase, alanine transaminase levels should be monitored and consider discontinuing if levels rise to greater than 10 times the upper limit of normal.[18]

Molnupiravir is a prodrug of ribonucleoside that has shown some antiviral activity in clinical trials and an EUA was issued in December 2021.[18,26] Molnupiravir was authorized for nonhospitalized patients of age 18 or older with mild to moderate COVID-19 within 5 days of symptoms and high risk of progression to severe COVID-19 for whom alternative therapies are not clinically appropriate.[18,31] The MOVe-OUT study was a large randomized, double-blinded controlled trial and the results showed reduced risk of hospitalization or death by 31% and reduced pulmonary complications.[32] The PANORAMIC open label trial showed that molnupiravir did not reduce frequency of COVID-19 hospitalizations or deaths in high-risk vaccinated patients versus usual care but did reduce the time to improvement of symptoms.[33]

The last recommended antiviral therapy, COVID-19 convalescent plasma (CCP), was initially an EUA therapy early during the pandemic with revision in 2022 and the treatment remains investigational.[34] Results from several large studies, however, did not show benefit.[35–37] COVID-19 CCP is human plasma collected from donors that have high titers of anti-SARS-CoV-2 antibodies. Current guidelines do not recommend for or against the use of CCP due to lack of supporting data; however, some panel members reported that they would use CCP in immunocompromised patients, particularly if the CCP was obtained from vaccinated donors who recently recovered with a similar variant.[18]

Immunomodulators

There are 3 main categories of immunomodulators currently recommended: systemic corticosteroids, anti–IL-6 receptor monoclonal antibodies, and janus kinase (JAK) inhibitors.

Corticosteroids are synthetic analogs of the hormones produced by the adrenal cortex and have multiple mechanisms of actions including anti-inflammatory and immunosuppressive effects along with other effects such as metabolic, electrolyte, central nervous system, and blood cell effects.[38] Dexamethasone is a glucocorticoid systemic steroid, and when administered, it binds through the glucocorticoid receptor leading to a reduction in proinflammatory cytokines, chemokines, and other enzymes involved in the inflammatory response. The RECOVERY randomized control trial showed that dexamethasone use of 6 mg daily for up to 10 days lowered 28-day mortality in hospitalized patients receiving respiratory support of oxygen or MV.[39] Other smaller sample studies have shown support for glucocorticoids such as hydrocortisone and methylprednisolone.[40–43] See **Table 2** for dosing recommendations.

Tocilizumab is a recombinant monoclonal antibody that is an IL-6 receptor antagonist.[44] IL-6 is responsible for proinflammatory cytokine release, and tocilizumab treats both the "cytokine storm" and also supports corticosteroid effects.[18,44] Studies have shown the most benefit in patients who are severely ill with COVID-19, on high-flow nasal cannula (HFNC) or noninvasive ventilation (NIV), or deteriorating rapidly on oxygen, or have a significant inflammatory response.[18,45,46] Tocilizumab was approved in 2022 by the FDA for hospitalized COVID-19 patents.[26]

Baricitinib is a JAK inhibitor and is hypothesized to block SARS CoV-2 from infecting the lungs with anti-inflammatory and antiviral effects.[18,47,48] The drug was approved by the FDA for EUA in late 2020 with full FDA approval in May 2022 for hospitalized patients requiring oxygen, NIV, MV, or ECMO.[26,49] The ACTT-2 study demonstrated that baricitinib plus remdesivir had superiority over remdesivir alone, including improved recovery time and 28-day mortality for patients on HFNC or NIV.[47]

Vilobelimab is an investigational monoclonal antibody that binds specifically to components of the complement system that contributes to inflammation and worsening of COVID-19.[18] It is under EUA only for treatment related to COVID-19 beginning April 2023.[18,26] The PANAMO study was a randomized multicenter controlled trial that showed a significant reduction in 28-day mortality in patients with MV.[50] An earlier trial had demonstrated safety in a smaller population of patients.[51]

There are an additional 4 therapies that are off-label uses of medications that are not FDA-approved for use in COVID-19 but are included in the National Institutes of Health guidelines based on ongoing research.[18] (see **Table 2**) Abatacept and infliximab are immunomodulators that are currently recommended as alternatives to either baricitinib or tocilizumab in hospitalized patients who require conventional oxygen, HFNC, or NIV in patients who are also receiving dexamethasone.[18] Both drugs were trialed in a large multiarm study comparing either drug to placebo and both drugs demonstrated a reduction in 28-day mortality.[52] Tofacitinib, a JAK inhibitor, or sarilumab, an IL-6 inhibitor, is recommended only if none of the preferred or alternative immunomodulator therapies are available or feasible and similarly should also be given with dexamethasone.[18] The STOP-COVID study showed decreased mortality or respiratory failure for patients taking Tofacitnib versus a placebo.[53] Sarilumab was studied as an IV formulation in the large REMAP-CAP trial and did show improved survival in 1 of the study arms.[54,55]

Anticoagulation

In the initial stages of the pandemic, it was unclear whether therapeutic anticoagulation was safe and would improve outcomes. Three large COVID-19 studies were integrated into a randomized controlled trial to examine outcomes of therapeutic anticoagulation versus usual care prophylaxis dosing.[56] While the trial was halted due to futility, the results in over 1000 patients demonstrated that therapeutic anticoagulation did not increase the probability of survival to discharge or number of days free of cardiovascular or respiratory organ support.[56] Additionally, there was an 89% probability of lower survival versus usual care prophylaxis dosing[56] (**Table 3**).

Oxygenation

Improving oxygenation is a primary goal during treatment due to the hallmark of progressive hypoxemia in COVID-19. Pulse oximetry (SpO2) is an indicator and not a direct measure of arterial oxygenation; however, it is the 1 component of oxygenation assessment that is readily available for continuous bedside monitoring.[57] Recent guidelines suggest a targeted goal SpO2 of 92% to 96% in patients with COVID-19.[18] Caution should be taken in patients with brown or black pigmented skin due to the risk for unrecognized hypoxemia.[58] A recent study in COVID-19 patients showed that SpO2

Table 3
Anticoagulation recommendations for hospitalized coronavirus disease 2019 patients

Clinical Criteria for Hospitalized Patients	Anticoagulant Therapy Recommendation
Admitted for reasons other than COVID-19 with high risk of progressing to severe COVID-19	Prophylactic heparin dosing (unfractionated or low molecular weight) for patients without an indication for therapeutic anticoagulation unless contraindicated.
Does not require oxygen but are at high risk of progressing to severe COVID-19	Prophylactic heparin dosing (unfractionated or low-molecular-weight) for patients without an indication for therapeutic anticoagulation unless contraindicated.
Requires minimal conventional oxygen	Therapeutic heparin (unfractionated or low molecular weight) dosing for nonpregnant patients with elevated D-dimer levels without increased bleeding risk. Prophylactic heparin (unfractionated or low-molecular-weight) dosing for all other patients without an indication for therapeutic anticoagulation
Requires high-flow nasal cannula, noninvasive ventilation, invasive mechanical ventilation, or extracorporeal membrane oxygenation	Prophylactic heparin dosing (unfractionated or low-molecular-weight) for hospitalized patients without an indication for therapeutic anticoagulation. For patients started on therapeutic heparin dosing (unfractionated or low-molecular-weight) in non-ICU setting and transferred to an ICU, recommend switching to prophylactic heparin dosing unless another indication for therapeutic anticoagulation.

Abbreviations: COVID-19, coronavirus disease 2019; ICU, intensive care unit.
Data from COVID-19 Treatment Guidelines Panel. Coronavirus disease 2019 (COVID-19) treatment guidelines. National Institutes of Health. 2023. Available at https://www.covid19treatment guidelines.nih.gov/. Accessed October 12, 2023.

significantly overestimated SaO2 in Black, Hispanic, and other ethnic minority patients compared with White patients.[59] Unrecognized hypoxemia in this study led to delayed therapy although there was no association with in-hospital mortality.[59] In patients with COVID-19 and acute hypoxemic respiratory failure (AHRF), oxygen is usually delivered using a nasal cannula, a face mask, or a non-rebreather mask and escalated to HFNC if the patient fails to respond or to NIV, if HFNC is unavailable.[18] HFNC delivers warm, humidified oxygen with a flow up to 70 L/minute and up to 100% fraction of inspired oxygen. A meta-analysis had shown prior to the pandemic that intubation rates are lower in patients who receive HFNC in AHRF.[60] The pandemic led to an increase in the use of HFNC in AHRF and reinforced the ease of use and benefits of HFNC in COVID-19.[61]

Awake prone positioning
A trial of awake prone positioning (APP) is recommended for patients with persistent hypoxemia when endotracheal intubation is not currently indicated.[18] Research has shown that early APP versus usual care in patients with AHRF in COVID-19 reduces the need for intubation.[62–67] Physiologically, APP appears to improve oxygenation by reducing dead space, respiratory rate, and work of breathing.[68] APP has been described in many studies, but in general, the procedure consists of an alert patient

Table 4
Current guideline recommendations for mechanical ventilation for acute respiratory distress syndrome and coronavirus disease 2019

	NIH Guideline[18]	ESICM Guideline[71]	SCCM Guideline[19]
Mechanical ventilation with moderate to severe ARDS and COVID-19	Recommend low tidal volume ventilation (VT 4–8 mL/kg of predicted body weight)	Same	Same
	Recommend targeting plateau pressure of<30 cm H2O	No information	Same
	Recommend conservative fluid strategy	No information	Same
	Recommend against routine use of nitric oxide	No information	Same
	Recommend using a higher PEEP strategy over lower PEEP strategy	Unable to make a recommendation for or against higher PEEP/Fio_2 strategy vs lower PEEP/Fio_2 strategy. Unable to make a recommendation for or against PEEP titration guided by respiratory mechanics compared to PEEP titration based on a standardized PEEP/Fio_2 table.	Same
	Recommend prone ventilation 12–16 hours/day with refractory hypoxemia despite optimal ventilation.	Recommend starting prone position early after intubation, after a period of stabilization and prone positioning for 16 consecutive hours or more.	Suggest prone ventilation 12–16 h over no prone ventilation.
	Recommend intermittent boluses of NMBAs or continuous NMBA infusion to facilitate protective lung ventilation as needed.	Unable to make a recommendation for or against the routine use of continuous NMBA.	Suggest using intermittent boluses of NMBAs over continuous NBMAs to facilitate protective lung ventilation. Suggest continuous NMBAs for up to 48 h for persistent dyssynchrony, need for deep sedation, or persistently high plateau pressures.

(continued on next page)

Table 4
(continued)

	NIH Guideline[18]	ESICM Guideline[71]	SCCM Guideline[19]
Rescue therapies	Recommend against using recruitment maneuvers; if used, recommend against the use of incremental PEEP recruitment maneuvers.	Recommend against use of prolonged high-pressure recruitment maneuvers. Suggest against routine use of brief high-pressure recruitment maneuvers.	Suggest using recruitment maneuvers over not using for hypoxemia despite optimizing ventilation.
	Recommend using an inhaled pulmonary vasodilator as a rescue therapy; if no rapid improvement in oxygenation, the treatment should be tapered off.	No information	Suggest a trial of inhaled pulmonary vasodilator as a rescue therapy in severe ARDS and hypoxemia despite optimization and other rescue therapies. If no rapid improvement in oxygenation, should be tapered off.
ECMO	There is insufficient evidence to recommend either for or against the use of ECMO.	Recommend that patients with severe ARDS due to COVID-19 should be treated with ECMO at an ECMO center adhering to management strategy similar to that of EOLIA trial.	Suggest using VV ECMO if available or referring to ECMO center for patient with refractory hypoxemia despite optimization, rescue therapies, and prone positioning.

Abbreviations: ARDS, acute respiratory distress syndrome; cm, centimeters; COVID-19, coronavirus disease 2019; ECMO, extracorporeal membrane oxygenation; ELOIA trial, extracorporeal membrane oxygenation for severe acute respiratory distress trial; ESICM, European Society of Intensive Care Medicine; Fio$_2$, fraction of inspired oxygen; mL, milliliters; NIH, National Institutes of Health; NMBA, neuromuscular blocking agents; PBW, predicted body weight; PEEP, positive end expiratory pressure; SCCM, Society of Critical Care Medicine; VT, tidal volume.
Data from Refs.[18,19,71]

who is able to assist with positioning and protect their airway while alternating positioning between prone, side lying, and supine with the head of the bed elevated for 30 minutes to 4 hours, 2 to 4 times a day.[69,70] The important differences between APP for nonintubated patients and traditional prone position for ARDS patients is the patient's ability to participate in positioning, lack of need for sedation or paralytics, frequency of position changes, and the ability to care for the patient in either an ICU or a non-ICU setting.

Mechanical ventilation
Many of the recommendations for MV are similar to guidelines for ARDS patients without COVID-19[18,19,71,72] (**Table 4**).

Prone positioning
The recommendation for prone positioning has been a strongly recommended evidence-based intervention for ARDS patients for over 10 years.[72,73] The increase in ARDS during the pandemic rose dramatically and led to rapid increase in prone positioning use with multiple protocols published to help prevent some of the more common complications including pressure injuries.[74–78] Current COVID-19 guidelines align with previous guidelines for proning of mechanically ventilated patients, recommending 12 to 16 hours of prone positioning for patients with refractory hypoxemia despite optimized ventilation.[18,19,71]

Box 1	
Laboratory work and other diagnostics	
Initial	• CBC
	• CMP
Consider	• ABG
	• Coagulation screen (PT, PTT, fibrinogen, D-dimer)
	• C-reactive protein
	• Ferritin
	• LDH
	• CK, CK-MB
	• Troponin
	• Blood and sputum cultures
	• ECG
	• CXR
Other testing	Based on possible therapeutics chosen or other patient conditions (See **Table2**: COVID-19 medications)

Abbreviations: ABG, arterial blood gas; CBC, complete blood count; CK, creatine kinase; CK-MB, creatine kinase-myocardial band; CMP, comprehensive metabolic panel; CXR, chest x ray; ECG, electrocardiogram; LDH, lactate dehydrogenase; PT, prothrombin time; PTT, partial thromboplastin time.

Data from American College Emergency Physicians. *ACEP COVID-19 Field Guide.* 2nd ed. American College Emergency Physicians. 2023. Available at: https://www.acep.org/corona/covid-19-field-guide/assessment/laboratory-abnormalities. Accessed October 22, 2023.

Extracorporeal membrane oxygenation

ECMO is a mechanical circulatory device that supports the heart or the heart and lungs.[79] Due to the increase in severe ARDS during the pandemic, there was an increase in the use for hypoxemic respiratory failure due to ARDS and COVID-19. Multiple guidelines have established criteria for ECMO and include maximizing traditional ARDS therapies, careful patient selection, and the use of experienced ECMO centers.[19,71,80,81] Findings from a recent large multicenter observational study suggested that in patients of age 60 years or older, the use of inotropes and vasopressors before ECMO, chronic renal failure, and time from intubation to ECMO greater than 4 days were all associated with higher mortality.[82] Current evidence is largely limited to ECMO in non-COVID-19 patients and further randomized control trials are needed to establish best practice in COVID-19 patients.[18]

Other Supportive Therapies

Treatment of patients with COVD-19 includes medical management, symptom management, infection control measures, and supportive therapies. These may include antipyretics for fever and pain, nutrition, appropriate hydration, decreasing risk for others with appropriate personal protective equipment, and preventing complications.[21] Monitoring such asSpO2 and cardiac monitoring should be implemented as indicated based on the patient's condition and severity of illness.

Recommended diagnostics including laboratory testing should be ordered based on COVID-19 diagnosis but also considering patient underlying conditions, severity of illness and possible therapeutics ordered (**Box 1**).

SUMMARY

The care and treatment of COVID-19 patients has considerably more evidence to guide practice than when the pandemic started. Therapeutics and management continue to evolve as higher level research, such as large randomized controlled trials, is done to answer many of the ongoing evidence-based practice questions. The SARS-CoV-2 virus also continues to mutate with possible impact on severity and transmission due to new variants. Access to updated guidelines and recommendations are essential. Every nurse should be aware of the resources in their health system along with the many health care associations that have made COVID-19 resources and research easily obtainable on their Web sites.

CLINICS CARE POINTS

- COVID-19 is caused by the RNA virus SARS-CoV-2 and is spread through respiratory secretions and droplets.
- COVID-19 infection can lead to multiorgan failure, most commonly leading to lung injury, AKI, and coagulopathy.
- COVID-19 patients are classified based on the severity of illness of mild, moderate, and severe to determine treatment modalities.
- While COVID-19 is no longer a public health emergency, many therapeutics remain under EUA with mandatory requirements to administer.
- The 3 main medication classes for COVID-19 consist of antivirals, immunomodulators, and anticoagulants.
- Mechanical ventilation interventions for COVID-19 patients with ARDS is similar to practice for non-COVID-19 ARDS patients.

- Ongoing research is needed to continue to determine evidence-based protocols for APP.

DISCLOSURE

The authors have nothing to disclose.

REFERENCES

1. Lim MS, Mcrae S. COVID-19 and immunothrombosis: pathophysiology and therapeutic implications. Crit Rev Oncol Hematol 2021;168:103529.
2. Triggle CR, Bansal D, Ding H, et al. A comprehensive review of viral characteristics, transmission, pathophysiology, immune response, and management of SARS-CoV-2 and COVID-19 as a basis for controlling the pandemic. Front Immunol 2021;12:631139.
3. Swenson KE, Swenson ER. Pathophysiology of acute respiratory distress syndrome and COVID-19 lung injury. Crit Care Clin 2021;37(4):749–76.
4. Murali R, Wanjari UR, Mukherjee AG, et al. Crosstalk between COVID-19 infection and kidney diseases: a review on the metabolomic approaches. Vaccines (Basel) 2023;11(2):489.
5. Beyerstedt S, Casaro EB, Rangel ÉB. COVID-19: angiotensin-converting enzyme 2 (ACE2) expression and tissue susceptibility to SARS-CoV-2 infection. Eur J Clin Microbiol Infect Dis 2021;40(5):905–19.
6. Montazersaheb S, Hosseiniyan Khatibi SM, Hejazi MS, et al. COVID-19 infection: an overview on cytokine storm and related interventions. Virol J 2022;19(1):92.
7. Zanza C, Romenskaya T, Manetti AC, et al. Cytokine storm in COVID-19: immunopathogenesis and therapy. Medicina (Kaunas) 2022;58(2). https://doi.org/10.3390/medicina58020144.
8. Fajgenbaum DC, June CH. Cytokine storm. N Engl J Med 2020;383(23):2255–73.
9. Hu B, Huang S, Yin L. The cytokine storm and COVID-19. J Med Virol 2021;93(1):250–6.
10. Narota A, Puri G, Singh VP, et al. COVID-19 and ARDS: update on preventive and therapeutic venues. Curr Mol Med 2022;22(4):312–24.
11. Mason RJ. Pathogenesis of COVID-19 from a cell biology perspective. Eur Respir J 2020;55(4):2000607.
12. Attaway AH, Scheraga RG, Bhimraj A, et al. Severe covid-19 pneumonia: pathogenesis and clinical management. BMJ 2021;372:n436.
13. Schenck EJ, Hoffman K, Goyal P, et al. Respiratory mechanics and gas exchange in COVID-19-associated respiratory failure. Ann Am Thorac Soc 2020;17(9):1158–61.
14. Tobin MJ, Laghi F, Jubran A. Why COVID-19 silent hypoxemia is baffling to physicians. Am J Respir Crit Care Med 2020;202(3):356–60.
15. Adamczak M, Surma S, Więcek A. Acute kidney injury in patients with COVID-19: epidemiology, pathogenesis and treatment. Adv Clin Exp Med 2022;31(3):317–26.
16. Zhou X, Cheng Z, Hu Y. COVID-19 and venous thromboembolism: from pathological mechanisms to clinical management. J Personalized Med 2021;11(12):1328.
17. Liu H, Wang Z, Sun H, et al. Thrombosis and coagulopathy in COVID-19: current understanding and implications for antithrombotic treatment in patients treated with percutaneous coronary intervention. Front Cardiovasc Med 2021;7:599334.

18. COVID-19 Treatment Guidelines Panel. Coronavirus disease 2019 (COVID-19) treatment guidelines. National Institutes of Health; 2023. Available at. https://www.covid19treatmentguidelines.nih.gov/. Accessed October 12, 2023.

19. Alhazzani W, Evans L, Alshamsi F, et al. Surviving Sepsis Campaign guidelines on the management of adults with coronavirus disease 2019 (COVID-19) in the ICU: first update. Crit Care Med 2021;49(3):e219–34.

20. Bhimraj A, Morgan RL, Shumaker AH, et al. Infectious Diseases Society of America guidelines on the treatment and management of patients with COVID-19. Infectious Diseases Society of America; 2023. Version 11.0.0. 2023. Available at. https://www.idsociety.org/practice-guideline/covid-19-guideline-treatment-and-management/. Accessed August 22, 2023.

21. World Health Organization. Clinical management of COVID-19: living guideline. 2023. Available at: https://www.who.int/publications/i/item/WHO-2019-nCoV-clinical-2023.2. Accessed August 21, 2023.

22. Guerin PJ, McLean AR, Rashan S, et al. Definitions matter: heterogenity of COVID-19 disease severity criteria and incomplete reporting compromise meta-analysis. PLOS Glob Public Health 2022;2(7):e0000561.

23. U.S. Food & Drug Administration. Emergency use authorization. 2023. Available at Emergency Use Authorization | FDA. Accessed September 2, 2023.

24. U.S. Food & Drug Administration. FAQs: What happens to EUAs when a public health emergency ends. 2023. . Available at FAQs: What happens to EUAs when a public health emergency ends? | FDA. Accessed September 2, 2023.

25. Phizer Laboratories. Highlights of prescribing information: Paxlovid. 2023. Available at labeling.pfizer.com/ShowLabeling.aspx?id=19599. Accessed August 21, 2023.

26. U.S. Food and Drug Administration. Coronavirus (COVID-19) drugs, . Food and drug administration. https://www.fda.gov/news-events/press-announcements/fda-approves-first-oral-antiviral-treatment-covid-19-adults. Accessed September 8, 2023.

27. Hammond J, Leister-Tebbe H, Gardner A, et al. Oral nirmatrelvir for high-risk, nonhospitalized adults with COVID-19. N Engl J Med 2022;386:1397–408.

28. Gilead. Highlights of prescribing information: Veklury. 2023. Available at veklury_-pi.pdf (gilead.com). Accessed August 21, 2023.

29. Beigel JH, Tomashek KM, Dodd LE, et al. Remdesivir for treatment of COVID-19 – final report. N Engl J Med 2020;383:1826–33.

30. Chokkalingam AP, Hayden J, Goldman JD, et al. Association of remdesivir treatment with mortality among hospitalized adults with COVID-19 in the United States. JAMA Netw Open 2022;5(12):e2244505.

31. Merck. Fact sheet for healthcare providers: emergency use authorization for lagevrio™ (molnupiravir) capsules. 2023. Available at molnupiravir-hcp-fact-sheet.pdf (merck.com). Accessed August 21, 2023.

32. Bernal AJ, da Silva G, Musungaie DB, Musungaie DB, et al. Molnupiravir for oral treatment of COVID-19 in nonhospitalized patients. N Engl J Med 2022;386:509–20.

33. Butler CC, Hobbs FD, Gbinigie OA, et al. Molnupiravir plus usual care versus usual care aloe as early treatment for adults with COVID-19 at increased risk of adverse outcomes (PANORAMIC): an open-label, platform-adaptive randomized controlled trial. Lancet 2023;401(10373):281–93.

34. U.S. Food and Drug Administration. Recommendations for investigational COVID-19 convalescent plasma. Food and Drug Administration 2022. Available at: https://www.fda.gov/vaccines-blood-biologics/investigational-new-drug-applications-

inds-cber-regulated-products/recommendations-investigational-covid-19-convalescent-plasma. Accessed September 21, 2023.

35. Writing Committee for the REMAP-CAP Investigators, Abdelrazik M, Abdi Z, et al. Effect of convalescent plasma on organ support-free days in critically ill patients with COVID-19: a randomized clinical trial. JAMA 2021;326(17):1690–702.

36. RECOVERY Collaborative Group, Abbas A, Abbas F, et al. Convalescent plasma in patients admitted to hospital with COVID-19 (RECOVERY): a randomised controlled, open-label, platform trial. Lancet 2021;397(10289):2049–59.

37. Begin P, Callum J, Jamula E, et al. Convalescent plasma for hospitalized patients with COVID-19: an open-label, randomized controlled trial. Nat Med 2021;27(11): 2012–24.

38. Hodgens A, Sharman T. StatPearls: corticosteroids. StatPearls Publishing; 2023. Available at: https://www.ncbi.nlm.nih.gov/books/NBK554612/. Accessed September 18, 2023.

39. The Recovery Collaborative Group. Dexamethasone in hospitalized patients with COVID-19. N Engl J Med 2021;384:693–704.

40. Dequin PF, Heming N, Meziani F, et al. Effect of hydrocortisone on 21-day mortality or respiratory support among critically ill patients with COVID-19: a randomized clinical trial. JAMA 2020;324(13):1298–306.

41. Angus DC, Derde L, Al-Beidh F, et al. Effect of hydrocortisone on mortality and organ support in patients with severe COVID-19: the REMAP-CAP COVID-19 corticosteroid domain randomized clinical trial. JAMA 2020;324(13):1317–29.

42. Corral-Gudino L, Bahamonde A, Arnaiz-Revillas F, et al. Methylprednisolone in adults hospitalized with COVID-19 pneumonia: an open-label randomized trial (GLUCOCOVID). Wien Klin Wochenschr [Central J Euro Med] 2021;133(7–8): 303–11.

43. Tang X, Feng YM, Ni JX, et al. Early use of corticosteroid may prolong SARS-CoV-2 shedding in non-intensive care unit patients with COVID-19 pneumonia: a multi-center, single-blind. randomized control trial Respiration 2021;100(2):116–26.

44. Abidi E, El Nekidy WS, Alefishat E, et al. Tocilizumab and COVID-19: timing of administration and efficacy. Front Pharmacol 2022;13:825749.

45. Salamar C, Han J, Yau L, et al. Tocilizumab in patients hospitalized with Covid-19 pneumonia. N Engl J Med 2021;384:20–30.

46. Genentech. Highlights of prescribing information: Actemra. 2022. Available at: actemra_prescribing.pdf (gene.com). Accessed August 21, 2023.

47. Kalil AC, Patterson TF, Mehta AK, et al. Baricitinib plus remdesivir for hospitalized adults with COVID-19. N Engl J Med 2021;384(9):795–807.

48. McLornan DP, Pope JE, Gotlib J, et al. Current and future status of JAK inhibitors. Lancet 2021;398(10302):803–16.

49. Eli Lilly and Company. Olumiant, baricitinib tablet, film coated. Update May 2022. Available at: These highlights do not include all the information needed to use OLUMIANT safely and effectively. See full prescribing information for OLUMIAN-T.OLUMIANT (baricitinib) tablets, for oral useInitial U.S. Approval: 2018 (lilly.com). Accessed August 21, 2023.

50. Vlaar AP, Witzenrath M, van Paassen P, et al. Anit-C5a antibody (vilobelimab) therapy for critically ill, invasively mechanically ventilated patients with COVID-19 (PANAMO): a multicentre, double-blind, randomized, placebo-controlled, phase 3 trial. Lancet Respir Med 2022;10(12):1137–46.

51. Vlaar AP, de Bruin S, Busch M, et al. Anti-C5a antibody IFX-1 (vilobelimab) treatment versus best supportive care for patients with severe COVID-19 (PANAMO):

an exploratory, open-label, phase 2 randomized controlled trial. Lancet Rheumatol 2020;2:e764–73.

52. O'Halloran JA, Ko ER, Anstrom KJ, et al. Abatacept, Cenicriviroc, or Infliximab for treatment of adults hospitalized with COVID-19 pneumonia. JAMA 2023;330(4): 328–99.

53. Guimaraes PO, Quirk D, Furtado RH, et al. Tofacitinib in patients hospitalized with COVID-19 pneumonia. N Engl J Med 2021;385(5):406–15.

54. REMAP-CAP Investigators. Interleukin-6 receptor antagonists in critically ill patients with covid-19. N Engl J Med 2021 Apr 22;384(16):1491–502.

55. Writing Committee for the REMAP-CAP Investigators, Higgins AM, Berry LR, et al. Long-term (180-day) outcomes in critically ill patients with COVID-19 in the REMAP-CAP randomized clinical trial. JAMA 2023;339(1):39–51.

56. The REMAP-CAP, ACTIV-4a, and ATTACC Investigators. Therapeutic anticoagulation with heparin in critically ill patients with COVID-19. N Engl J Med 2021; 385(9):777–89.

57. Lucas A, Bond D. Oxygen saturation monitoring with pulse oximetry. In: Johnson KA, editor. AACN procedure manual for high acuity, progressive, and critical care. 8th edition. St. Louis, MO: Elsevier Saunders; 2023. p. 135–42.

58. Sjoding OL, Dickson RP, Iwashyna TJ, et al. Racial bias in pulse oximetry measurement. N Engl J Med 2020;383(25):2477–8.

59. Fawzy A, Wu TD, Wang K, et al. Clinical outcomes associated with overestimation of oxygen saturation in pulse oximetry in patients hospitalized with COVID-19. JAMA Netw Open 2023;6(8):22330856.

60. Ni YN, Luo J, Yu H, et al. The effect of high-flow nasal cannula in reducing the mortality and the rate of endotracheal intubation when used before mechanical ventilation compared with conventional oxygen therapy and noninvasive positive pressure ventilation. A systematic review and meta-analysis. Am J Emerg Med 2018;36(2):226–33.

61. Genecand L, Agoritsas T, Ehrensperger C, et al. High-flow nasal oxygen in acute hypoxemic respiratory failure: a narrative review of the evidence before and after the COVID-19 pandemic. Front Med 2022;9:1068327.

62. Tian ET, Gatto CL, Amusina O, et al. Assessment of awake prone positioning in hospitalized adults with COVID-19. JAMA Intern Med 2022;182(6):612–21.

63. Li J, Luo J, Pavlov I, et al. Aware prone positioning for non-intubated patients with COVID-19-related acute hypoxaemic respiratory failure: a systematic review and meta-analysis. Lancet Respir Med 2022;10:573–83.

64. Weatherald J, Parhar KK, Duhalib ZA, et al. Efficacy of awake prone positioning in patients with covid-19 related hypoxemic respiratory failure: systematic review and meta-analysis. BMJ 2022;379:e071966.

65. Siddiqui A, Ochani S, Cheema HA, et al. Awake prone positioning for patients with COVID-19 and acute respiratory failure: a meta-analysis. Crit Care Med 2023;51(1):S472.

66. Musso G, Taliano C, Paschetta E, et al. Mechanical power delivered by noninvaive ventilation contributes to physio-anatomical and clinical responses to early versus late proning in COVID-19 pneumonia. Crit Care Med 2023;51(9):1185–200.

67. Cheema HA, Siddiqui A, Ochani S, et al. Awake prone positioining for non-intubated COVID-19 patients with acute respiratory failure: a meta-analysis of randomised controlled trials. J Clin Med 2023;12:926.

68. Lehnigue S, Allardet-Servent J, Ferdani A, et al. Physiologic effects of the awake prone position combined with high-flow nasal oxygen on gas exchange and work

of breathing in patient with severe COVID-19 pneumonia: a randomized cross-over trial. Crit Care Explor 2022;4(12):e0805.

69. Seckel MA. Awake self-prone positioning and the evidence. Crit Care Nurse 2021;41(4):76–9.

70. Allicock KA, Coyne D, Garton AN, et al. Awake self-prone positioning: implementation during the COVID-19 pandemic. Crit Care Nurse 2021;41(5):23–33.

71. Grasselli G, Calfee CS, Camporota L, et al. ESICM guidelines on acute respiratory distress syndrome: definition, phenotyping and respiratory support strategies. Intensive Care Med 2023;49:727–59.

72. Guerrin C, Reignier J, Richard J, et al. Prone positioning in severe acute respiratory distress syndrome. N Engl J Med 2013;368:2159–68.

73. Fan E, Del Sorbo L, Goligher EC, et al. An official American Thoracic Society/European Society of Intensive Care Medicine/Society of Critical Care Medicine clinical practice guideline: mechanical ventilation in adult patients with acute respiratory distress syndrome. Am J Respir Crit Care Med 2017;195(9):1253–63.

74. Binda F, Galazzi A, Marelli F, et al. Complications of prone positioning in patients with COVID-19: a cross sectional study. Intensive Crit Care Nurs 2021;67:103088.

75. Makic MB. Prone position of patients with COVID-19 and acute respiratory distress syndrome. J Perianesth Nurs 2020;35(4):437–8.

76. Ryan P, Fine C, DeForge C. An evidence-based protocol for manual prone positioning of patients with ARDS. Crit Care Nurse 2021;41(6):55–61.

77. Morata L, Vollman K, Rechter J, et al. Manual prone positioning in adults: reducing the risk of harm through evidence-based practices. Crit Care Nurse 2023;43(1):59–66.

78. Vollman KM, Mitchell DM. Prone positioning for acute respiratory distress syndrome patients. In: Johnson KA, editor. AACN procedure manual for high acuity, progressive, and critical care. 8th edition. St. Louis, MO: Elsevier Saunders; 2023. p. 143–56.

79. Moutray K, Ebberts M. Extracorporeal membrane oxygenation. In: Johnson KA, editor. AACN procedure manual for high acuity, progressive, and critical care. 8th edition. St. Louis, MO: Elsevier Saunders; 2023. p. 122–34.

80. ELSO COVID-19 Working Group. Extracorporeal life support organization COVID-19 interim guidelines. April 12, 2000. Available at: https://www.elso.org/portals/0/files/pdf/elso%20covid%20guidelines%20final.pdf. Accessed October 19, 2023.

81. Tonna JE, Abrams D, Brodie D, et al. Management of adult patients supported with venovenous extracorporeal membrane oxygenation (VV ECMO): guideline from the extracorporeal life support organization (ELSO). ASAIO J 2021;67(6):601–10.

82. Lorusso R, De Piero ME, Mariana S, et al. In-hospital and 6-month outcomes in patients with COVID-19 supported with extracorporeal membrane oxygenation (EuroEMCO-COVID): a multicentre, prospective observational study. Lancet Resp Med 2023;11:151–62.

Challenges and Solutions to Patient Safety During a Pandemic

Susan M. Holland, EdD, MSN, RN, NEA-BC

KEYWORDS

- Safety • Risk • Communication • COVID-19

KEY POINTS

- The US Public Health system response was robust.
- Communication was key in the COVID-19 pandemic.
- Centralized response in hospitals promoted patient safety.
- Unintended patient safety impacts resulted from the COVID-19 pandemic response.

BACKGROUND

Although COVID-19 was a novel disease that very little was known about at the start of the pandemic, the complex and far-reaching public health system in the United States truly helped to minimize transmission and maximize communication between government agencies (federal, state, and local), hospitals, health care professionals, and ultimately, the general public.

The very existence of such an advanced public health system that already existed in the United States and had processes in place to manage public health emergencies in general was key to providing safe care to patients who contracted COVID-19, to protect frontline staff, and to protect the public.

Certainly, there are areas for improvement, but without such a structure already in place, the overall response to the pandemic would not have been as coordinated and efficient. For example, the existence of the Department of Health and Human Services[1] in the federal government includes many operating divisions under its umbrella, including the Centers for Disease Control and Prevention (CDC),[2] Centers for Medicare & Medicaid Services (CMS),[3] and the National Institutes of Health (NIH).[4] These are just a few of the federal divisions that helped prevent an even greater loss of life during the COVID-19 pandemic.

Within each of these divisions are more specialized branches, such as the National Center for Emerging and Zoonotic Infectious Diseases[5] (within the CDC), the

Beth Israel Deaconess Medical Center, 330 Brookline Avenue, Boston, MA 02215, USA
E-mail address: sholland@bidmc.harvard.edu

Crit Care Nurs Clin N Am 36 (2024) 323–336
https://doi.org/10.1016/j.cnc.2024.02.001
ccnursing.theclinics.com

Emergency Preparedness and Response Operations[6] (within CMS), and the National Institute of Allergy and Infectious Diseases[7] (within NIH). Of course, there are many more agencies, divisions, and branches of both the federal and state governments that were involved in the COVID-19 pandemic response, and these are just a few examples to highlight the complex and well-designed public health system that was already in existence. Despite the communication with health care systems and the public in general, including the sharing of the science behind masking, social distancing, and eventually vaccination, there was still a component of skepticism among the public about trusting health care leaders and fear of harm from being vaccinated. In a piece looking historically at the reaction of society to other public health threats, such as Ebola, Jones[8] explained that history suggests that society is at risk from exaggerated fears and misplaced priorities. For example, someone who lives in the United States may have worried about contracting Ebola even though the risk was very small, whereas that same person may not take precautions and get vaccinated against influenza, which is an illness that is known to kill thousands of people annually.[8,9] The purpose of this article is to identify the unique challenges that caregivers faced during the COVID-19 pandemic regarding patient safety and describe strategies that were implemented that also included efforts to ensure staff safety and well-being so they could remain working and caring for these patients.

CENTRALIZED RESPONSE AS A KEY TO SAFETY

Just as the federal, state, and local governments responded to the COVID-19 pandemic, so did hospitals and in particular critical care units. Early on, hospitals began a central response to the crisis, recognizing that this required a coordinated process. In most hospitals, there may be a type of command center in cases of internal or external disasters. The team members who are part of the command center collect and organize information, coordinate the hospital's response, and are responsible for communicating with hospital staff. When it became clear that the number of patients with COVID-19 was increasing, hospitals often stopped admitting patients for "elective" procedures, recognizing that the term "elective" does not mean "not needed." By doing this, it freed up space in hospitals so that patients with COVID-19 could be cared for while also allowing for the redeployment of staff from areas such as the operating room to help in other patient care areas.[10,11]

The members of a centralized command center must include at a minimum the hospital administrator or designee, a nurse leader, a physician leader, and a leader of other operations, such as maintenance and facilities. Of course, in larger hospitals, there may be more individuals as part of this team, including a representative from Patient Safety. In a situation such as COVID-19, the Director of Infection Control and/or an Infectious Disease physician would also be a key member of the command center team.

COMMUNICATION

Because new knowledge was being learned rapidly, and to ensure that there were clear, coordinated communications throughout the hospital, a method for communicating information "out" to the hospital, as well as a way to communicate "into" the command center was needed. By centralizing communications and coming to some type of consensus or democratization of crisis communication, staff anxiety may be reduced, coordination may be improved, and a safer workplace and safer environment of care may be fostered.[12]

To maintain the safest environment for patients, staff, and visitors, it was necessary for there to be clear and coordinated communication from hospital leadership to all staff members. In addition, all essential areas needed to be represented at leadership meetings, such as nursing, medicine, pharmacy, dietary, environmental services/housekeeping, and so forth, so that key issues could be shared and briefly discussed, and decisions made then or soon after the meeting. Communication of decisions and dissemination of information can serve as "lifelines" for frontline workers and managers. Through honest, clear, and coordinated communication, hospital leadership is showing that they value the input from all staff, take concerns seriously, and want to make the best decisions in the best interest of staff, patients, and others. Transparency and honesty are key to help build and sustain trust.

SAFETY OF WORKFORCE

If one conceptually applies Maslow's Hierarchy of Needs Theory[13] in the context of the ability of hospitals to care for patients who are admitted with COVID-19, one may first consider the environment of care, and more importantly, the workforce. Toward the beginning of the pandemic, there were so many unknowns, including a definitive understanding about how the infection was spread. Nurses and other health care workers were often not only anxious about this and what it meant for them but also concerned about what they could bring home to their loved ones after caring for these patients. These fears were evident as preparation was occurring, often before a hospital was caring for any patients with COVID-19. Although all of the answers were not there, hospital leaders needed to ensure that they responded with the current knowledge at that time, in a coordinated manner. It was very important to respond therapeutically in these situations and listen to the fears of nurses and other team members, and although no one had all of the answers, and there was very little known about COVID-19, being present and empathizing with colleagues could be very supportive. Atkinson and colleagues[14] identified specific leadership practices that were most impactful on a hospital's performance and resiliency during the COVID-19 crisis management. Examples of these practices included "consistent communication and coordination with hospitals and organizations in the local community" and "leadership practices that demonstrated transparency and supportiveness, as well as a collaborative hospital culture."[14(p21)]

While planning to care for patients who will be admitted to the hospital with COVID-19, there must be a focus on the workforce itself. Although most individuals may have chosen the field of health care for altruistic reasons, they are still concerned about their own safety and the safety of their loved ones. Listening to these concerns from health care workers, providing reassurance when possible, being transparent and honest, and providing resources/support are all necessary to help sustain a high performing team and resiliency.[14] If a health care worker is worried about their parents or children, for example, it may be difficult for them to focus on the task at hand, such as preparing to care for this influx of patients.

There were times when hospitals as well as federal, state, and local governments provided resources that helped make it easier for some of the frontline care providers to go to work. In some places, college dormitories were used as spaces to house health care workers who were concerned about caring for patients with COVID-19 and then going home to loved ones, fearing that they could spread the illness to them.[15] Later, as it was learned how the virus was actually spread, these fears decreased, but some health care workers chose to continue to use this housing so they would be closer to the hospital and be able to work more hours.

Siddique and colleagues[16] described the work experiences during the pandemic, and the most challenging included decreased staffing, and increase in workload, and feeling that they were unable to take time off owing to the COVID-19 vaccine side effects (when nurses were needed so much). The physical exhaustion of these nurses cannot be overstated. Working long shifts wearing an N95 mask along with other personal protective equipment (PPE) created a more uncomfortable, hot, and humid working environment.[17–21] There were less opportunities to take a moment to have a sip of water from the break room (as one would need to doff PPE first) and even less opportunities to break for a longer period.

Although caregivers wore PPE when caring for patients with COVID-19, there was still a risk of transmission of COVID-19 to staff. This was a greater concern at the beginning of the pandemic when less was known about the mechanisms for transmission and when most hospitals implemented a system of reusing PPE out of necessity because of a lack of supplies (ie, the same N95 mask used by one staff member for many days).[17–21] Consolidating care and limiting the number of times a health care provider was exposed to a patient with COVID-19 was a consideration in planning for intensive care unit (ICU) nurses to be able to care for a greater number of patients with the assistance of other non-ICU nurses. In addition to decreasing the risk of transmission, this was also a way to conserve PPE.[22]

Other examples of interventions to provide care safely included transforming larger non-ICU inpatient units into ICUs to expand the capacity for caring for patients requiring critical care.[23] Unfortunately, many medical/surgical units do not have windows in their doors to view patients. It was critical to visualize these ICU patients who were now being cared for in non-ICU settings (ie, to help monitor for signs of an increase in a patient's Richmond Agitation Sedation Scale,[24] prevent accidental extubation, and prevent patient falls). To allow for visualization of patients while the doors to rooms were closed for infection control safety, the doors to patient rooms were reconfigured so they had a window installed. This allowed easier visualization of the patients if the nurse did not need to enter to complete some assessments or perform an intervention. Other creative methods were used, such as using long intravenous (IV) tubing so that the pump could be kept outside of patient rooms to decrease the frequency of entering the patients' rooms and therefore decreasing the amount of times a health care worker was exposed and allowed conservation of PPE.[22,23]

The Institute for Healthcare Improvement (2020) published a tool with evidence-based recommendations for "psychological PPE that can help protect staff mental health in the face of extreme working conditions such as natural disasters, terrorist attacks, and previous pandemics."[25(p2)] Other ways leaders supported health care workers' well-being during COVID-19 included providing proactive support to manage fear and anxiety in daily work, providing opt-out mental health and well-being support, and creating opportunities for staff to reconnect meaning and purpose in their work.[26] Another approach to help protect health care workers was peer support; however, there needs to be awareness of the potential for these peer supporters to become overwhelmed themselves, particularly as they will also likely be working in extreme conditions, such as caring for patients during a pandemic. Godfrey and colleagues[27] found high levels of emotional exhaustion among peer supporters in COVID-19 units.

For most health care organizations in the United States, universal masking of staff and visitors was the norm, but health care providers did become ill at times with COVID-19 whether the exposure was while at work or from being in the community.[28] This of course created challenges for staffing on top of existing staffing demands; however, by having clear guidelines for staff members to refer to and a process to follow, helped to prevented the transmission of COVID-19 to patients and other health care workers. Some nurses struggled with the desire to care for patients in this un-precedented pandemic while not feeling well and being required to stay home until a certain point, and in one study, 80% of medical providers continued to work despite having influenza-like illness.[29–31]

SCARCITY OF SUPPLIES

It was a priority to keep the workforce free from infection from COVID-19. In order to care for patients with COVID-19, and to protect the health care worker as well as other patients, it was necessary for providers to wear an N95 mask, or alternative if avail-able. Early in the pandemic, it became evident that there was going to be a shortage of the N95 masks in most hospitals.[16,17] Many hospitals likely had some type of stock-pile of N95 masks because, for years, there were emergency drills to respond to a flu pandemic. However, these stockpiles were not enough. Also, because typically when one hospital was searching for a particular piece of PPE, others were as well, causing the local, state, and ultimately federal stockpiles to dwindle.

Creative solutions, such as storing one's mask in a container for future use, were implemented, and the reuse of masks was essential. There were novel methods tried to extend the usage of these masks, whereby the originally disposable mask was sent to be cleaned, returned, and reused by the same staff member. During the pandemic, there was temporary approval given by the OSHA (Occupational Safety and Health Administration) that these masks could be reused by the same health care worker.[32] Understandably, nurses and others were very concerned about this practice for their own safety as well as for the safety of their loved ones.

Throughout the pandemic there were nationwide shortages of various patient care items and medications.[33] This inevitably led to either a change in practice or the use of a piece of equipment that was not the typical device that staff were used to. One could understand how this could create a risk for patient safety; however, the only interven-tion that seemed plausible at the time was to provide clear and coordinated commu-nication and education regarding these changes. An analysis completed by the Healthcare Association of New York State's standing Statewide Steering Committee on Quality Initiatives reported that the availability of critical supplies and equipment during the COVID-19 pandemic included items such as PPE (masks, gowns, gloves, and eye protection), ventilators, COVID-19 testing supplies, oxygen needs in "new" units, oxygen adapters, pulse oximeters, negative pressure rooms, dialysis equip-ment, and drug supplies for certain classes of drugs.[33,34]

During the COVID-19 crisis, hospitals did not have enough negative pressure rooms to accommodate caring for all of the patients encountered, and portable HEPA filters may have been used, or in many cases, an entire unit would be designated as caring for patients with COVID-19, and N95 masks and other PPE were needed to be worn by staff whenever they were in that unit. This presented a great many challenges for staff members who had to wear PPE for long periods of time, such as dehydration, facial ulcers, and discomfort in general.[19–21]

COORDINATION OF PATIENT CARE IN THE CRITICAL CARE UNITS

It became evident that there was a shortage of nurses and other members of the health care team during the COVID-19 pandemic. Many nurses chose to retire if they were eligible, left inpatient nursing to pursue another specialty, or decided to leave organi-zations to become a travel nurse and take advantage of this opportunity, which was beneficial financially.[35,36] Also, health care workers started becoming ill with COVID-19, further depleting the workforce. All of these things contributed to an increased workload on the nurses and other health care providers who remained and cared for patients with COVID-19 or other inpatients.

This gap in staff was somewhat filled most often by travel nurses, or in some cases, the state government may have made emergency provisions to allow senior nursing students to work as "graduate nurses" under the supervision of a Registered Nurse (RN). In addition, nurses from other inpatient units who did not have ICU experience underwent a tailored training and were often assisting ICU nurses in caring for an ICU patient assignment. All of these creative methods were implemented to improve the number of nurses available to staff a unit; nevertheless, this came with potential risks to patient safety. However, in a review of literature, there was no association between the use of travel nurses and patient outcomes, but rather negative outcomes may have been more associated with staffing and the general work environment.[36,37]

Because of this restructuring of patient care assignments and formation of new care teams, it was key that the flow of communication between ICU nurses and these non-ICU nurses was clear and flowed both ways for the safety of patients. The same requirements for communication were conveyed when working with "proning teams," who often included perioperative nursing staff who possessed expertise in patient positioning, including positioning patients prone, which was one of the therapeutic care interventions provided to patients with COVID-19.[22,23] Again, it was essential that communication was clear, flowing in both directions, and questions were encouraged.

Coordination of these changes in processes and practices through the command center was necessary to account for the appropriate space or environment of care, education, supplies, and/or equipment that would be needed and the numbers and specialties of staff members to support this new unit. For many hospitals, it was essential to have Human Resources assisting with tracking/accounting for employees in addition to direct managers. Health care workers were redeployed based on their competency and past experience to assist in COVID-19 care units, to assist in ICUs, or to become part of "proning teams," and so forth. Often a restructuring of traditional nurse-to-patient ratios was done because of the limited amount of specialized ICU nurses or medical/surgical inpatient nurses where the ICU/OR medical /surgical nurse would have an assignment of patients greater than would be typical, but would also be assigned a nurse or other health care provider to assist that nurse. Orientation for these "helper" nurses was abbreviated and focused on what they "needed to know" or "needed to do" as part of their helper role. The other portions of the nurse's role, including traditional assessments and directing care, was completed by the primary nurse.

There were other examples of restructuring the traditional organization of the patient care team in COVID-19 ICUs. Emory Healthcare in Atlanta, Georgia established general ratios and team roles in the care of patients in ICUs during the COVID-19 pandemic. Although nurses cared for more patients than typical, there was a team of health care providers assisting with aspects of care for that group of patients and aligned the care delivery model with the Quality and Safety Education for Nurses competencies.[23,38–40]

NURSING LEADERSHIP

Nurse leaders had to adapt quickly to the changing landscape of nursing care of patients with COVID-19 in critical care environments, including ensuring competence and providing a supportive environment where nurses feel safe to ask questions or ask for help of experienced ICU nurses. Compassion fatigue was found to be significantly higher in nurses who worked more than 50 hours per week and in nurses who faced ethical problems and ethical decisions that were not being supported.[40] Brimhall and colleagues[41] reported that "leaders who understand employees' unique needs, express confidence in employees' abilities and encourage employees to share their ideas, create inclusive and trusting work environments that encourage psychological safety and ultimately help reduce reported medical errors."[41(p120)] Because there was little that could be considered predictable or controlled during the pandemic, strong nursing leadership was necessary to sustain teams and support health care workers.

The COVID-19 crisis of course was not only occurring when a health care provider was at work, it impacted all areas of life. High-quality work relationships among health care workers during the COVID-19 crisis where relational coordination was evident positively influenced the resilience of these staff members at work and at home. Examples of relational coordination at work includes timely communication, shared goals, problem-solving communication, sharing of knowledge, schedule control, and mutual respect.[42] One way for health care leaders to influence an employee's feeling of schedule control is to consider individual employee's different needs and preferences (ie, Sally may request Tuesdays off and prefer not to work more than two 12-hour shifts in a row, whereas Tim may prefer to work three 12-hour shifts in a row). Certainly, it may not always be possible to accommodate these needs and requests, but making an effort to do so is an example of personalized support.

INTERVENTIONS AND UNINTENTIONAL IMPACTS TO PATIENT SAFETY
Prioritization of Patient Care

Even with these non-ICU nurses assisting with care, there were times nurses were required to prioritize the care that they were providing, again focusing on life-sustaining treatment first. The risks of these changes could have included a decrease in the frequency of assessment of IV sites and a risk of tubing disconnection among other things. Also, the patients' compromised health status alone created a situation where they were more susceptible to acquiring a pressure injury, so any decrease in the frequency of turning and repositioning could hasten the development of this type of wound. In addition, a lack of staff training and the length of time that it took to don PPE when patients were on precautions were found to have contributed to patient falls during the COVID-19 pandemic.[43]

Potential for Health Care Inequities

It is known that health inequities exist in health care, and one must be aware that there is a connection between patients' social needs and poor health outcomes.[44] Jarrett and colleagues[34] explained that "longstanding inequities in healthcare were exposed during the pandemic, leading to greater spread within at-risk communities, increasing the likelihood of an overwhelmed healthcare delivery system."[34(p475)] It is important to acknowledge this and proactively prevent inequity of care, particularly in times of crisis.

Visitor Safety

During the height of COVID-19, all visitation of patients was restricted, and an exception may be made if a patient was transitioning to comfort care or hospice. During these times, there were many stories about the emotional pain endured by patients and loved ones who were not allowed to visit. This was done to protect the visitors from exposure to COVID-19 from their loved one and others, but also contributed to harm. For example, there were circumstances such as when 2 siblings needed to decide who was going to be the one person to visit their father at the end of his life and say goodbye. Not only were these family members and patients suffering because of this, but the nurses and other caregivers involved were also suffering and experiencing moral distress. When these situations occurred, it was often the nurse who was the lone voice, required to share the rules with patients and families.

A qualitative study exploring visitors' perceptions of the visitation restrictions during COVID-19 revealed themes of "advocacy, communication, emotional upheaval, human factors, isolation, and abandonment."[45] Dudeck and colleagues[46] identified defining attributes of family presence during COVID-19 and acknowledged that nurses can act as surrogates in the absence of a patient's support person. A proposed definition of family presence during times when visitation is restricted includes the following:

Family members (mothers, parents, relatives, or significant others) being there or with the patient, either physically, virtually, or through a surrogate, when the patient is admitted to the hospital during this challenging time. Although families may not be physically present at the bedside, seeing the patient on a virtual window convinces them that their loved ones are being cared for and will not simply disappear. This unconventional patient-and-family-centered approach can also be used to identify a subjective advocate who may serve as surrogate for the patient's social support or network. Remote visitation can be implemented through various technological platforms, such as an iPad, laptop, or smartphones.[46(p143)]

Patient Safety Reports/Incident Reports

If nurses and other health care providers needed to prioritize patient care because of volume and acuity and did not have time to document all they would have liked to on patients, it was likely that they were not able to enter all of the incident reports/patient safety reports that they could have during the COVID-19 pandemic. This has unfortunately led to a gap in information where the data that hospitals collect, including near misses and learning opportunities, are likely not complete. During the COVID-19 pandemic, Idilbi and colleagues[47] found that nurses who were female had more experience, worked the morning shift or were academics, had higher perceptions of a patient safety culture, were more likely to report a near-miss event as well as a higher rate of the reporting of events. In addition, the themes that emerged when exploring the intentions of nursing staff to report a near-miss event during COVID-19 were as follows: underreporting of events, staffing, physical and mental overload, and poor departmental organization.[47] There were patient-safety reports/incident reports entered; however, it is difficult to know if caregivers were able to report everything that they normally would during the COVID-19 pandemic. Health care teams responded to problems or challenges during the COVID-19 pandemic with thoughtful and creative interventions.

However, these interventions may have had unintentional negative impacts on patient safety. Examples of these unintentional impacts on patient safety are outlined in **Table 1**.

DISCUSSION

Before the worldwide COVID-19 pandemic, there were articles and drills to try to prepare health care professionals and others for a pandemic that was predicted to occur at some point. In 2019 (before the pandemic), Aaron E. Glatt, MD,[2] who was the chairman of the Department of Medicine and Hospital Epidemiology at Mount Sinai–South Nassau Communities Hospital, wrote a commentary in a business journal about

Table 1
Interventions and unintentional impacts on patient safety

Problem	Intervention	Challenge/Unintentional Impact
Nursing shortage	Travel nurses and less experienced RNs	Potential for lack of resources and support in a crisis situation
Influx of patients with COVID-19 requiring ICU care	Cancel "elective" surgeries/procedures and redeploy non-ICU nurses to help in ICU	An "elective" procedure does NOT mean, "not needed"; potential for a delay in a procedure that caused an unsafe situation for another patient; ensuring adequate training and clarity of roles
Need to limit staff exposures to COVID-19	Prioritize care; complete care during blocks of time	Potential for missed nursing interventions; potential for an increase in patient falls
Increase in volume and acuity of patients with COVID-19	Prioritize care; decrease the amount of required documentation	Potential for missed nursing interventions; likely underreporting of events in patient safety reporting systems
Limit visitor exposures to COVID-19	Not allow visitors (except for 1 person at end of life)	Psychological harm to patient and family; moral distress for nurse and other care providers and may increase the potential for health care inequities if a patient relied on a family member to advocate for them
Product shortages	Redesign of processes and use of other manufacturers' products	Potential for error because of knowledge deficit to new process or using different equipment

the 1919 flu pandemic and reported how the CDC has been involved in creating a global influenza surveillance system that included 114 World Health Organization[48(p115)] members, stating that,

"Vaccination remains the single best and most important instrument in our efforts to prevent both epidemic and pandemic influenza. The enormous loss of life due to flu one hundred years ago remains a stark and forbidding lesson. Fighting the next pandemic cannot be done alone by public health officials. Each of us has a responsibility to be vaccinated."[49]

Hall[50] reflected on the 2009 H1N1 pandemic and how it helped pharmacists prepare and train for similar situations in the future, including how using pharmacies during a flu pandemic could significantly reduce the time that was needed to immunize adults. In addition, a Memorandum of Understanding toolkit for public health and pharmacies was created in preparation for a flu pandemic. No doubt that this toolkit, among other preparatory documents and workflows, helped in the nationwide and worldwide response to the COVID-19 pandemic, preparing for the development of a vaccine.

In addition, the Healthcare Association of New York State's standing Statewide Steering Committee on Quality Initiatives "prepared [a] report using multiple performance improvement methodologies to identify risks and opportunities in current structures, processes, and outcomes, and establish root causes and develop recommendations."[34] This report identified 8 categories: staffing, equipment, environment, trusted information, competency, education and training, communication, and human factors. Each category was analyzed and included recommendations for improvement, including how hospitals and health systems should work together to procure much needed supplies, such as PPE, during COVID-19 for the best value and to avoid stockpiling and collaborate to determine where equipment should be sent based on the greatest need. There were many recommendations for county, state, and federal policymakers, such as assuring that PPE and equipment supply chains have adequate stockpiles to avoid shortages in the future, and along with this, how warehousing should be affordable so these inventories can be stored.[34]

Finally, the importance of leadership, communication, and safety cannot be overlooked.

The participation of senior or executive leaders in a hospital is essential in establishing an effective command center that essentially focuses on coordinating communication and removing barriers in the emergency management process. Middle managers, such as Nurse Managers, and others who had daily interactions with staff members, such as Nurse Specialists or Educators, were key in communicating both problems and strategies to the command center so coordinated responses or decisions could be made. Both formal and informal leaders in patient care units were key to the successful implementation of emergency management plans responding to the COVID-19 pandemic. This event demonstrated the importance of investing in the development of nursing leadership throughout a hospital, which may include supporting those pursuing advanced degrees in Nursing Administration or Nursing Education and succession planning.

The consideration of safety in all aspects of responding to the COVID-19 pandemic was essential. Every member of the care team needed to consider what was best and safest for these patients being cared for in nontraditional ICUs or other adaptive environments. All caregivers were aware of the potential risk of being infected themselves with COVID-19 while caring for these patients and the potential of bringing this virus home unknowingly. The amount of anxiety and stress experienced by all team members particularly at the beginning of the pandemic and when there were shortages in PPE cannot be understated. Despite this, and working long shifts, wearing PPE, during a nursing shortage, the nurses and others continued to report to work to care for these patients for many months and years.

SUMMARY AND FUTURE WORK

The health care community will continue to learn about the true impact of this worldwide pandemic on patient safety over time by examining hospital processes, quality indicators, patients' feedback, staff experiences, and outcomes. Nursing research is key to exploring the topic of patient safety among many other aspects of the response to the COVID-19 pandemic.

Hospital leaders must acknowledge that one of the greatest challenges facing health care management following the COVID-19 crisis includes "the centrality of human resource constraints (amidst increasing demand), the necessity of collaboration (amidst competition), and a need to reconsider the approach to leadership (utility of humility)."[51(p185)]

CLINICS CARE POINTS

- Hospitals must react quickly and begin a central response to any crisis, recognizing that it requires a coordinated process.
- Many hospitals use a command center approach in cases of internal or external disasters and include specific team members in order to collect and organize information, coordinate the hospital's response, and communicate with hospital staff.
- Hospitals must consider not only the safety of patients and staff within the hospital environment but also the impact that a disaster (such as a pandemic) may have on the families and loved ones of employees. Leaders must consider how they may provide support to employees so that they are able to come to work to care for patients.
- Most hospitals canceled elective procedures during the COVID-19 pandemic. However, an "elective procedure" does NOT mean that it is not needed, and there may be consequences in delaying procedures or tests that may result in patient harm.
- Hospitals eliminated or limited patient visitation to protect the visitors, patients, staff, and community. However, in doing so, this caused emotional harm or distress on occasion to patients, loved ones, and staff members particularly during end-of-life care.

DISCLOSURE

The author does not have any commercial or financial conflicts of interest.

REFERENCES

1. United States Department of Health and Human Services. Available at: https://www.hhs.gov/. [Accessed 3 January 2024].
2. Centers for Disease Control (CDC). Available at: https://www.cdc.gov/. [Accessed 3 January 2024].
3. Centers for Medicare and Medicaid (CMS). Available at: https://www.cms.gov/. [Accessed 3 January 2024].
4. National Institutes of Health (NIH). Available at: https://www.nih.gov/. [Accessed 3 January 2024].
5. National Center for Emerging and Zoonotic Infectious Diseases (NCEZID). Centers for Disease Control (CDC). 2024. Available at: https://www.cdc.gov/ncezid/index.html. [Accessed 3 January 2024].
6. Emergency preparedness & response operations. Centers for Medicare and Medicaid (CMS). 2023. Available at: https://www.cms.gov/about-cms/what-we-do/emergency-response. [Accessed 3 January 2024].
7. National Institute of Allergy and Infectious Diseases. National Institutes of health (NIH). Available at: https://www.niaid.nih.gov/. [Accessed 3 January 2024].
8. Jones DS. History in a crisis- lessons for COVID-19 (perspective). N Engl J Med 2020;382:18.
9. Disease burden of flu. Centers for disease control (CDC). 2023. Available at: https://www.cdc.gov/flu/about/burden/index.html#print. [Accessed 3 January 2024].
10. Mehta A, Awuah WA, Ng JC, et al. Elective surgeries during and after the COVID-19 pandemic: case burden and physician shortage concerns. Ann Med Surg (Lond) 2022;81:104395.

11. US hospitals, patients cancel elective surgery as coronavirus spreads. Reuters. 2020. Available at: https://www.reuters.com/article/us-health-coronavirus-usa-surgery-idUSKBN2133SK/. [Accessed 4 January 2024].

12. Hayirli T, Stark N, Hardy J, et al. Centralization and democratization: managing crisis communication in health care delivery. Health Care Manag Rev 2023;48: 292–300.

13. Maslow AH. A theory of human motivation. Psychol Rev 1943;50:370–96. Available at: https://www.researchhistory.org/2012/06/16/maslows-hierarchy-of-needs/?print=1. [Accessed 4 January 2024].

14. Atkinson M, Biddinger P, Chughtai MA, et al. Assessing health care leadership and management for resilience and performance during crisis: the HERO-36. Health Care Manag Rev 2024;49:14–22.

15. Brown provides short-term residence hall housing to front-line personnel fighting COVID-19. Brown University News; 2020. Available at: https://www.brown.edu/news/2020-04-21/residence. [Accessed 4 January 2024].

16. Siddique S, Rice S, Bhardwaj M, et al. Health care organization policies for employee safety and COVID-19 pandemic response: a mixed methods study. J Occup Environ Med 2023;65(1). https://doi.org/10.1097/JOM.0000000000002741.

17. US Food and Drug Administration (FDA). (2020). Face shields and other barrier emergency use authorizations (EUAs), personal protective equipment EUAs. 2023. Available at: https://www.fda.gov/medical-devices/covid-19-emergency-use-authorizations-medical-devices/personal-protective-equipment-euas#respirators. [Accessed 4 January 2024].

18. US Food and Drug Administration (FDA). (2023). N95 respirators, surgical masks, face masks, and barrier face coverings, personal protective equipment for infection control. 2023. Available at: https://www.fda.gov/medical-devices/personal-protective-equipment-infection-control/n95-respirators-surgical-masks-face-masks-and-barrier-face-coverings#s3. [Accessed 4 January 2024].

19. Wan X, Lu Q, Sun D, et al. Skin barrier damage due to prolonged mask use among healthcare workers and the general population during the COVID-19 pandemic: a prospective cross-sectional survey in China. Dermatology 2022; 238:218–25.

20. Baker TL, Greiner JV, Vesonder M. SARS-CoV-2 safety: guidelines for shielding frontline nurses. Nursing 2021;51(3). https://doi.org/10.1097/01.NURSE.0000733932.88107.44.

21. Manookian A, Nayeri ND, Shahmari M. Physical problems of prolonged use of personal protective equipment during the COVID-19 pandemic: a scoping review. Nurs Forum 2022;1–11. https://doi.org/10.1111/nuf.12735.

22. Hearvin S. COVID-19: every day innovations for the management of COVID-19 patients. American Hospital Association; 2020. www.aha.org/covid19. [Accessed 4 January 2024].

23. Geyer LT, Bennett SG, Atkins WJ, et al. Innovation amid pandemic. Journal for Nurses in Professional Development 2021;38(1):19–23.

24. Ely EW, Truman B, Shintani A, et al. Monitoring sedation status over time in ICU patients: reliability and validity of the Richmond Agitation-Sedation Scale (RASS). JAMA 2003;289(22):2983–91.

25. Psychological PPE. Promote health care workforce mental health and well-being. Institute for Healthcare Improvement; 2020. Available at: https://www.ihi.org/resources/tools/psychological-ppe-promote-health-care-workforce-mental-health-and-well-being. [Accessed 4 January 2024].

26. Laderman M, Perlo J. Industry voices- 3 actions to support healthcare workers' well-being during COVID-19. Institute for Healthcare Improvement, Fierce Healthcare 2020. Available at: https://www.fiercehealthcare.com/hospitals-health-systems/industry-voices-3-actions-to-support-healthcare-workers-well-being-during. [Accessed 4 January 2024].

27. Godfrey KM, Kozar B, Morales C, et al. The well-being of peer supporters in a pandemic: a mixed-methods study. Joint Comm J Qual Patient Saf 2022;48(9). Available at: https://www.sciencedirect.com/journal/the-joint-commission-journal-on-quality-and-patient-safety/vol/48/issue/9.

28. Baker C. Revised order requiring face coverings in public places-COVID-19 order No. 55. Commonwealth of Massachusetts. 2020. Available at: ///H:/A%20personal/CC%20clinics%20NA/Revised%20Face%20Coverings%20Order%20No.%2055.pdf. [Accessed 4 January 2024].

29. Preston-Suni K, Celedon MA, Cordasco KM. Patient safety and ethical implications of health care sick leave policies in the pandemic era. Joint Comm J Qual Patient Saf 2021;47:10. Accessed January 4, 2024.

30. Tartari E, Saris K, Kenters N, et al, International Society of Antimicrobial Chemotherapy Infection and Prevention Control ISAC-IPC Working Group. Not sick enough to worry? Influenza-like symptoms and work-related behavior among healthcare workers and other professionals: results of a global survey. PLoS One 2020. Available at: https://journals.plos.org/plosone/article?id=10.1371/journal.pone.0232168. [Accessed 4 January 2024].

31. Webster RK, Liu R, Hall I, et al. A systematic review of infectious illness presenteeism: prevalence, reasons and risk factors. BMC Publ Health 2019;19. https://doi.org/10.1186/s12889-019-7138-x. Accessed January 4, 2024.

32. Enforcement guidance for respiratory protection and the N95 shortage due to the coronavirus disease 2019 (COVID-19) pandemic. Archived Occupational Safety and Health Administration (OSHA). 2020. Available at: https://www.osha.gov/laws-regs/standardinterpretations/2020-04-03. [Accessed 4 January 2024].

33. Ranney ML, Griffeth V, Jha AJ. Critical supply shortages- the need for ventilators and personal protective equipment during the covid-19 pandemic. N Engl J Med 2020;382(41). https://doi.org/10.1056/NEJMp2006141.

34. Jarrett M, Garrick R, Gaeta A, et al. Pandemic preparedness: COVID-19 lessons learned in New York's hospitals. Joint Comm J Qual Patient Saf 2022;48(9). https://doi.org/10.1016/j.jcjq.2022.06.002. Accessed January 4, 2024.

35. 2020. Fact sheet: nursing shortage. American association of colleges of nursing (AACN). 2020. Available at: https://www.aacnnursing.org/news-data/fact-sheets/nursing-shortage. [Accessed 4 January 2024].

36. National Sample Survey of Registered Nurses (NSSRN). Health workforce. Health resources & services administration (HRSA). 2018. https://data.hrsa.gov/topics/health-workforce/nursing-workforce-survey-data. [Accessed 4 January 2024].

37. Weerdt V, Peck C, Tracy J, et al. Travel nurses and patient outcomes: a systematic review. Health Care Manag Rev 2023;48:352–62. Accessed January 4, 2024.

38. Kennedy E, Kennedy P, Hernandez J, et al. Understanding redeployment during the COVID-19 pandemic: a qualitative analysis of nurse reported experiences. SAGE Open Nurs; 2022. https://doi.org/10.1177/23779608221114985. Accessed January 4, 2024.

39. QSEN Institute competencies. Quality and safety education for nurses Institute. Available at: https://www.qsen.org/competencies. [Accessed 4 January 2024].

40. Gurdap Z, Cengiz Z. Compassion fatigue and ethical attitudes in nursing care in intensive care nurses during the COVID-19 pandemic. J Nurs Care Qual 2023; 38(4):312–8. Accessed January 4, 2024.

41. Brimhall K, Tsai YC, Eckardt R, et al. The effects of leadership for self-worth, inclusion, trust, and psychological safety on medical error reporting. Health Care Manag Rev 2023;48:120–9. Accessed January 4, 2024.

42. Ali H, Gittell J, Deng S, et al. Relationships and resilience at work and at home: impact of relational coordination on clinician work-life balance and well-being in times of crisis. Health Care Manag Rev 2023;48:80–91. Accessed January 4, 2024.

43. Venema D, Hester A, Clapper K, et al. Description and implications of falls in patients hospitalized due to COVID-19. J Nurs Care Qual 2023. https://doi.org/10.1097/NCQ.0000000000000733. Accessed January 4, 2024.

44. Peretz P, Shapiro A, Santos L, et al. Social determinants of health screening and management: lessons at a large, urban academic health system. Joint Comm J Qual Patient Saf 2023;49:6–7. Available at: https://www.sciencedirect.com/journal/the-joint-commission-journal-on-quality-and-patient-safety/vol/49/issue/6. [Accessed 4 January 2024].

45. Knight SL, Robinson R, Stinson C. No visitors: family perceptions of separation from hospitalized loved ones. Dimens Crit Care Nurs 2023;42:6. Accessed January 4, 2024.

46. Dudeck S, Hibler E, Gill K, et al. A concept analysis of family presence during COVID-19. Dimens Crit Care Nurs 2023;42:3. Accessed January 4, 2024.

47. Idilbi N, Dokhi M, Malka-Zeevi H, et al. The relationship between patient safety culture and the intentions of the nursing staff to report a near-miss event during the COVID-19 crisis. J Nurs Care Qual 2023;3(3):264–71.

48. World health organization (WHO). 2024. Available at: https://www.who.int/. [Accessed 4 January 2024].

49. Glatt AE. Dr Glatt: the flu pandemic of 1919 continues to cast a long shadow. Long I Bus News 2019. Available at: https://libn.com/2019/02/18/glatt-the-flu-pandemic-of-1919-continues-to-cast-a-long-shadow/. [Accessed 4 January 2024].

50. Hall DH. Pandemic vaccine planning: lessons learned and preparing for the future. Available at: Pharm Times 2017; https://www.pharmacytimes.com/view/pandemic-vaccine-planning-lessons-learned-and-preparing-for-the-future. [Accessed 4 January 2024].

51. Gifford R, Van de Baan F, Westra D, et al. Through the looking glass: confronting health care management's biggest challenges in the wake of a crisis. Health Care Manag Rev 2023;48:185–96. Accessed January 4, 2024.

Impacts of the COVID-19 Pandemic on Newly Licensed Critical Care Nurses

Angela Renkema, MPH, BSN, RN, NPD-BC, CV-BC, CPH,
Kelly Gallagher, MSN, RN, NPD-BC, NEA-BC*

KEYWORDS

- Transition to practice programs • Nurse Residency Program • New graduate nurses
- COVID-19 pandemic • Critical care

KEY POINTS

- The COVID-19 pandemic has increased the number of newly licensed registered nurses (NLRNs) hired into critical care areas.
- Turnover for critical care NLRNs has mirrored trends throughout the United States in the last few years. The NLRNs in critical care who began nursing in 2020 and 2021 saw an increase in turnovers in these years.
- Understanding why NLRNs are leaving is integral to sustaining, supporting, and reducing turnover. As reflected in the data, NLRNs leaving organizations due to "a job representing a different experience" increased by 5% from 2018 to 2021.
- NLRNs starting in 2020 and 2021 are less satisfied than NLRNs who started in 2018.
- Organizations must engage and support NLRNs throughout their first year of practice and beyond through Nurse Residency Programs and professional development opportunities.

INTRODUCTION

Nursing has been significantly impacted by the COVID-19 pandemic. Newly licensed registered nurses (NLRNs), especially those in critical care, were among those most affected. Interruptions and significant alterations in academia, clinical rotations, precepted experiences, and transition to practice programs impacted nearly all NLRNs. This article focuses on the pandemic's impacts on critical care NLRNs, the subsequent changes in the nursing workforce demographic, and the role of a Nurse Residency Program (NRP) in supporting NLRNs' transition to practice and improving outcomes.

Nurse Residency Program, Vizient, Inc., Chicago, IL, USA
* Corresponding author. 433 West Van Buren Street, Suite 805, Chicago, IL 60607.
E-mail address: Kelly.Gallagher@vizientinc.com

Crit Care Nurs Clin N Am 36 (2024) 337–352
https://doi.org/10.1016/j.cnc.2024.01.006
0899-5885/24/© 2024 Elsevier Inc. All rights reserved.
ccnursing.theclinics.com

BACKGROUND

The COVID-19 pandemic had a profound impact on all health care professionals including NLRNs. In fact, in a 2021 study, Ulrich and colleagues found that 67% of nurses reported they plan to leave their current position in the next 3 years.[1] Current literature describes the pandemic's impact on NLRNs including changes in prelicensure educational shifts from in-person classroom and clinicals to virtual classes, canceled capstone projects, decreased opportunities to practice skills and procedures, and limited clinical rotations with increased simulation-based learning.[2–5] These experiences, added to an already stressful time in which NLRNs who were acclimating to a new environment, became more overwhelming due to the addition of the COVID-19 pandemic.[6] NLRNs experienced vulnerability, uncertainty, and a need to adapt to changing policies and work environments during their first months of practice.[4,7] During the COVID-19 pandemic, NLRNs participating in an NRP described lower self-reported patient safety scores and commitment scores than those who participated in NRPs before the pandemic.[8]

Although literature describing the experiences of NLRNs during the pandemic exists, this program evaluation and comprehensive literature review adds to the literature focusing on hiring trends, experiences, and turnover of NLRNs in the critical care setting. Critical care nurses were particularly affected as they were on the frontline providing care to the most severely ill patients. Many experienced role frustration and challenging work environments. These nurses also faced emotional experiences such as fear, anxiety, exhaustion, stress, and the need to manage social stigma during various waves of the pandemic.[9,10] As a result, leaders from the Vizient/American Association of Colleges of Nursing (AACN) Nurse Residency Program sought to understand COVID-19s impacts on critical care NLRNs participating in the United States-wide NRP through a program evaluation analysis.

The Vizient/AACN NRP is a 12-month transition to practice program to increase NLRN retention rates, by supporting participants to develop skills necessary to improve decision-making, enhance clinical nursing leadership practices, and promote the incorporation of research-based evidence into practice.[11] Because hospitalizations were higher for adults compared with children during the first year of the pandemic,[12] we also sought to understand if there were differences on impacts of the NLRNs hired in adult critical care units compared with pediatric critical care units.

The purpose of this program evaluation is to understand how the NLRN nursing workforce changed during the COVID-19 pandemic for both adult and pediatric critical care NLRNs. This is a program evaluation, and therefore, not subject to institutional review board (IRB) approval. Previously, the University of North Carolina Chapel Hill IRB reviewed the evaluation structure and tools for the Vizient/AACN NRP and determined not to be human subjects' research.

DATA ANALYSIS

To understand the impact of the COVID-19 pandemic on NLRNs employed in critical care areas, data were evaluated for NLRNs who entered the NRP between 2018 and 2022. NLRNs who entered the NRP in 2018 completed the NRP before the pandemic. Data from 2018 served as a baseline for comparison.

- Some NLRNs who entered the NRP in 2019 completed the NRP before the start of the pandemic, whereas others were still enrolled in the NRP when the pandemic began.

- NLRNs who entered the NRP in 2020 may have experienced COVID-19-related interruptions or alterations in the later portions of their educational programs, and all were enrolled in the NRP during the pandemic. Data from this period demonstrated the impact during the initial stages of the pandemic.
- NLRNs who entered the NRP in 2021 experienced the impacts of both their nursing education and NRP.
- Demographic data for NLRNs who entered the program in 2022 are included in the analysis; however, survey data are not since these NLRNs are still in the process of completing a 12-month NRP in 2023 (at the time of publication submission).

The demographic and survey data were extracted from the Vizient/AACN NRP database, which is a secure, online database.[13] Organizations that actively participated in the NRP at the beginning of 2018 and maintained their involvement throughout the years analyzed (2018–2022) were included in the evaluation. This approach was implemented to ensure consistency when comparing data across different years by controlling for the number of organizations involved.

On hire, the site coordinator at the hiring institution determines an NLRNs assigned unit and enters the NLRNs demographic and unit information into the Vizient/AACN NRP database. **Table 1** indicates the types of units included stratified by pediatric or adult units for the analysis.

The site coordinator enters turnover data into the Vizient/AACN NRP database and selects the reason why the NLRN left their position. Turnover calculations were based on the year in which the NLRN started. For example, if an NLRN started in July 2018, and left the position in February 2019, the turnover would be attributed to 2018. Turnover for each year was analyzed for a 1-year period, defined as the period from the NLRNs first day in the NRP to day 365. Turnovers were reported as percentages based on the number of NLRNS who left their position divided by the total number of NLRNs in the year. Turnovers were further classified as either unavoidable or avoidable.

To understand the new nurse's experiences, NLRNs complete surveys on start, at 6 months and 12 months after starting the NRP. Surveys were completed via a secure online platform. Before completing the initial surveys, NLRNs must accept an attestation acknowledging that completed surveys can be used to analyze their transition into practice and that their survey responses can be used for research purposes. NLRNs were provided with the option to decline participation and were not required to complete the surveys. All survey responses were included in the analysis including those of NLRNs who left their positions before completion of the NRP and those who may have not completed all the surveys during the NRP.

Table 1
Adult critical care and pediatric critical care unit analysis groups

Adult Critical Care	Pediatric Critical Care
Cardiac/Heart/Vascular Critical Care Unit	Pediatric ICU Inpatient Unit
Medical ICU Inpatient Unit	Pediatric Intermediate Unit
Medical/Surgical ICU Inpatient unit	Neonatal ICU Inpatient Unit
Medical/Surgical Intermediate Unit	Neonatal Intermediate Unit
Neurology/Neurosurgical ICU inpatient unit	
Surgical ICU inpatient unit	

Data extracted from the database were analyzed using SAS version 9.4 (SAS Institute Inc). Hire and turnover data were analyzed using percentages, and percentage change was calculated. NLRN survey data were analyzed using the Mann–Whitney U test, with statistical significance set at $\alpha = 0.05$.

Two survey instruments are used to evaluate NLRN self-reported comfort with various aspects of practice and their overall satisfaction in nursing. These instruments include the Casey-Fink Graduate Nurse Experience Survey (CFGNES) and the Vizient/ AACN NRP Progression Survey (Progression Survey). The CFGNES was developed to assess NLRNs' experience as they transition into practice. The content validity of the tool was established by a review of nursing professional development practitioners and nursing directors. The survey focuses on the level of comfort and confidence in nursing skills and their organizational experience.[14] CFGNES patient safety domain and the CFGNES support domain were selected in this evaluation to understand the NLRNs experience and provide insight into turnover trends. For these questions, NLRNs were asked to rate themselves on a 4-point Likert scale of strongly disagree (1) to strongly agree (4). All questions require a response to submit the survey. The Cronbach's alpha for these two domains is 0.73 and 0.84, respectively.[15]

The Progression Survey was developed by the Vizient/AACN NRP to assess the NLRNs development in additional areas to the CFGNES.[13] The survey was developed by content experts from nursing academia, NRP coordinators, and nursing researchers. Areas were identified, and questions were developed from existing surveys and content experts. Once questions were developed, NLRNs reviewed the questions for fit and readability. The questions were piloted, and an exploratory factor analysis was completed. Overall, there are six domains in the Progression Survey and an assessment of self-reported competency level. To understand the satisfaction of the NLRNs, their self-reported competency level, and insight into turnover trends, three domains were analyzed: satisfaction and commitment, dissatisfaction, and self-reported competency. For the satisfaction and commitment domain and the dissatisfaction domain, response options are on a Likert scale of 1 (strongly disagree) to 4 (strongly agree). Responses to each question were required. The self-assessment for competency was on a scale of 0 (novice) to 10 (fully competent), where whole numbers were required. Internal validity with Cronbach's alpha is 0.92 (satisfaction and commitment) and 0.78 (dissatisfaction).

RESULTS

There were 272 organizations included in the analysis, including 17 that had missing organizational characteristics. **Table 2** depicts the organizational characteristics of the sample. Hiring trends, demographic information, turnover data, and survey data were analyzed.

Hiring Trends

Fig. 1 shows the number of NLRNs hired over the analysis years from the selected units. At baseline, in 2018, there 5528 NLRNs and 9065 at the conclusion of data analysis in 2022 (only organizations that were participating in the program in 2018 and all years until end date analysis in 2022) resulting in a 63.9% increase in hiring. In the 5 years of data analyzed across the 272 Vizient member organizations included in this analysis, 35,872 NLRNs were hired directly into critical care areas. **Fig. 2** shows the percent change in hiring trends between the adult and pediatric critical care areas over the evaluation period. Adult critical care areas demonstrated the most consistent increases in hiring. Pediatric critical care areas had small increases in hiring during

Table 2
Organizational characteristics

Category	Percentage
Types of organization	
Academic Medical Center	21.6%
Ambulatory Setting	0.4%
Community Hospital	36.9%
Rural Hospital	3.5%
Teaching Hospital	37.7%
Unionized	
No	82.4%
Yes	17.7%
American Nurses Credentialing Center (ANCC) Magnet Recognition Program	
No	59.2%
Yes	40.8%
ANCC Pathway to Excellence Program	
No	89.8%
Yes	10.2%
Nurse Residency Program Accreditation	
No	64.7%
Yes	35.3%

Note: Seventeen organizations had missing organizational characteristics were not included in this table and were included in the data analysis.

2020 and 2021, with a sharp increase in 2022 to 83.14% over the 2018 baseline period. **Table 3** provides the number of hires each year. Medical/surgical intermediate units had the highest number of hires in 2019 to 2021, and the second highest number of hires in 2018 and 2022. To understand how the pandemic impacted hiring, the percent change of hires each year was compared with the 2018 baseline year (**Fig. 3**). Since the pandemic did not begin until 2020, the pandemic did not exert any influence on hiring; however, its early impact may be evident in the survey data and turnover rates among NLRNs who were enrolled in the NRP between 2019 and

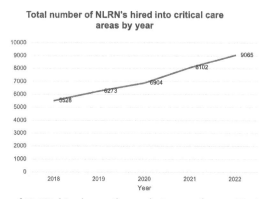

Fig. 1. The number of NLRNs hired over the analysis years from critical care units.

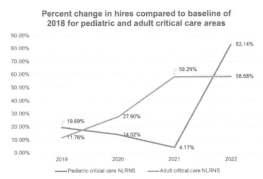

Fig. 2. The percent change in hiring trends between adult and pediatric critical care areas. Compared to 2018 baseline.

the onset of the pandemic. In 2020, all the adult critical care and intermediate units had at least a 13% increase in hiring from the baseline year of 2018, except for the surgical intensive care unit (ICU), which had a 5.8% increase in hires. The neonatal ICU and pediatric ICU followed the same trends as the adult critical care areas, with an increase in hires of 12.74% and 26.51%, respectively. In 2020, there were two units who had decreases in hiring when compared with the baseline year. These units were the neonatal intermediate unit and the pediatric intermediate unit.

Demographic Information

To continue to understand the impact of COVID-19 on the critical care NLRNs, demographic variables of age, degree, and grade point average (GPA) were analyzed. Although small shifts in percentages were noted over the years, meaningful changes were not noted. See **Table 4** for further details.

Turnover Data

Because the NRP first seminar date is used as day 1 for purposes of evaluating turnover rates, it is not an exact measure of first-year turnover. NLRNs may not be enrolled in their first NRP seminar until 1 to 3 months into practice; therefore, these rates most likely reflect turnover beyond the first year.

Turnover was divided into two categories: unavoidable and avoidable. Unavoidable reasons include reasons which an organization cannot control, such as death or NCLEX-RN failure. Examples of avoidable reasons include leaving for different job opportunities and leaving for a shorter commute. **Table 5** shows trends in the turnover data from 2018 to 2021. Avoidable turnover rates from 2018 to 2021 increased by 4.46%, and unavoidable turnover rates increased marginally by 0.28%. Turnover in NLRNs in the critical care area has mirrored trends throughout the United States in the last few years. The NLRNs in critical care who began nursing in 2020 and 2021 saw an increase in turnovers in these years.

In examining turnover reasons, there were shifts in responses for critical care NLRNs. **Table 6** highlights the turnover reasons that had notable percentage shifts from 2018 to 2021 for critical care NLRNs. The percent of overall turnovers decreased in the category of "relocating out of area" from 2018 to 2021. In 2018, 20.4% of critical care NLRN turnovers were due to relocating out of area; in 2021, the rate decreased to 15.9%. Another contributor to turnover that decreased was "unsatisfactory performance." In 2018, 13.4% of critical care NLRN turnovers were due to unsatisfactory performance, whereas in 2021 this decreased to 7.2%.

Table 3
The number and percent[a] of newly licensed registered nurses hired into critical care units by year

Unit Type	2018 N (%)	2019 N (%)	2020 N (%)	2021 N (%)	2022 N (%)
Medical Surgical ICU Inpatient Unit	727 (13.2%)	737 (11.8%)	822 (11.9%)	1040 (12.8%)	1322 (14.6%)
Pediatric ICU Inpatient Unit	430 (7.8%)	473 (7.5%)	544 (7.9%)	437 (5.4%)	791 (8.7%)
Neonatal ICU Inpatient Unit	636 (11.5%)	823 (13.1%)	717 (10.4%)	731 (9.0%)	1239 (13.7%)
Cardiac/Heart/Vascular Critical Care Unit	1029 (18.6%)	1182 (18.8%)	1275 (18.5%)	1625 (20.1%)	1738 (19.2%)
Medial ICU Inpatient Unit	621 (11.2%)	616 (9.8%)	742 (10.8%)	925 (11.4%)	932 (10.3%)
Medical/Surgical Intermediate Unit	918 (16.6%)	1275 (20.3%)	1552 (22.5%)	1842 (22.7%)	1534 (16.9%)
Neonatal Intermediate Unit	28 (0.5%)	31 (0.5%)	17 (0.3%)	24 (0.3%)	63 (0.7%)
Neurology/Neurosurgical ICU Inpatient Unit	690 (12.5%)	708 (11.3%)	782 (11.3%)	924 (11.4%)	787 (8.7%)
Pediatric Intermediate Unit	104 (1.9%)	107 (1.7%)	88 (1.3%)	56 (0.7%)	101 (1.1%)
Surgical ICU Inpatient Unit	345 (6.2%)	321 (5.1%)	365 (5.3%)	498 (6.2%)	558 (6.2%)
Total Number of NLRNs	5528	6273	6904	8102	9065

[a] Percentage indicates the NLRNs hired into the specific unit compared with all critical care units for that year.

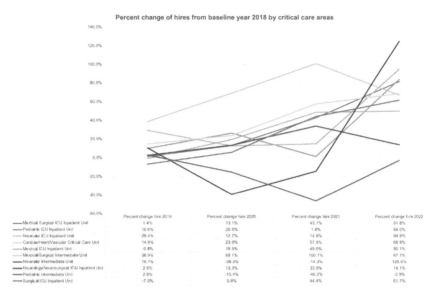

Percent change of hires from baseline year 2018 by critical care areas

	Percent change hire 2019	Percent change hire 2020	Percent change hire 2021	Percent change hire 2022
Medical Surgical ICU Inpatient Unit	1.4%	13.1%	43.1%	81.8%
Pediatric ICU Inpatient Unit	10.0%	26.5%	1.6%	84.0%
Neonatal ICU Inpatient Unit	29.4%	12.7%	14.9%	94.8%
Cardiac/Heart/Vascular Critical Care Unit	14.9%	23.9%	57.9%	68.9%
Medical ICU Inpatient Unit	-0.8%	19.5%	49.0%	50.1%
Medical/Surgical Intermediate Unit	38.9%	69.1%	100.7%	67.1%
Neonatal Intermediate Unit	10.7%	-39.2%	-14.3%	125.0%
Neurology/Neurosurgical ICU Inpatient Unit	2.6%	13.3%	33.9%	14.1%
Pediatric Intermediate Unit	2.9%	-15.4%	-46.2%	-2.9%
Surgical ICU Inpatient Unit	-7.0%	5.8%	44.4%	61.7%

Fig. 3. Trends in percent change of hires. Compared to 2018 baseline.

There was an increase in turnovers related to "obtained a position representing a different job experience." In 2018, only 10.4% of critical care NLRN turnovers were related to this reason; however, in 2021, 15.9% of critical care NLRN turnovers were related to this reason. In critical care NLRNs who were hired in 2020 and left organizations, 4% were listed as "leaving due to a pandemic or crisis"; for critical care NLRNs hired in 2021, this decreased to 0.8%. In 2020, a new category was added

Table 4
Critical care newly licensed registered nurse demographics

Demographics	2018 N (%)	2019 N (%)	2020 N (%)	2021 N (%)	2022 N (%)
Age (mean, median)[a]	25.8 (24)	25.8 (24)	25.8 (24)	25.9 (24)	25.9 (24)
Degree received					
Bachelors	4118 (74.5%)	4772 (76.2%)	5178 (75%)	6063 (74.8%)	6592 (72.7%)
Associates	1169 (21.2%)	1252 (20%)	1381 (20%)	1682 (20.8%)	2050 (22.6%)
Other	16 (0.3%)	17 (0.3%)	27 (0.4%)	10 (0.1%)	23 (0.3%)
Diploma	65 (1.2%)	66 (1.2%)	66 (1%)	101 (1.3%)	101 (1.1%)
Masters	160 (2.9%)	166 (2.7%)	252 (3.7%)	246 (3%)	299 (3.3%)
GPA[b]					
Not recorded	351 (6.4%)	2 (0.0%)	0	0	0
3.5 and above	2743 (49.6%)	3465 (55.2%)	4025 (58.3%)	4731 (58.4%)	5311 (58.6%)
3.0–3.49	2156 (39%)	2487 (39.7%)	2544 (36.9%)	3014 (37.2%)	3307 (36.5%)
2.5–2.99	256 (4.6%)	280 (4.5%)	314 (4.6%)	338 (4.2%)	409 (4.5%)
2.0–2.49	11 (0.2%)	22 (0.4%)	18 (0.3%)	18 (0.2%)	28 (0.3%)
Below 2.0	11 (0.2%)	17 (0.3%)	3 (0.0%)	1 (0.0%)	10 (0.1%)

[a] Outliers of less than 18 and greater than 70 removed.
[b] GPA was not required for reporting until 2020.

Table 5
Turnovers for critical care newly licensed registered nurses by year

Turnover Reasons	2018 Critical Care NLRNs	2019 Critical Care NLRNs	2020 Critical Care NLRNs	2021 Critical Care NLRNS
Unavoidable Reasons	0.16%	0.16%	0.36%	0.44%
Avoidable Reasons	9.97%	9.29%	13.47%	14.43%

titled "travel nurse." There are no baseline data to compare to for 2018; however, the reason "travel nurse" accounted for 3.3% of turnovers in critical care NLRNs who started in 2020 and increased to 3.8% of critical care NLRNs who started in 2021. To understand the academic impacts for critical care NLRNs, NCLEX-RN failure turnovers were examined. In 2018, "failed NCLEX" made up 0.5% of turnovers, and in 2019, 0.3% of turnovers. This increased in 2020 to 0.8% and in 2021 to 1.6% of all critical care NLRN turnovers were due to "failed NCLEX."

Self-Reported Newly Licensed Registered Nurse Survey Results

To help further understand the experience of NLRNs entering practice during the COVID-19 pandemic, domains from the surveys completed by NLRNs were analyzed in the Progression Survey (satisfaction and commitment, dissatisfaction, and self-assessment of competency domains) and the CFGNES (support and patient safety domains). The Mann–Whitney U test, with statistical significance of $\alpha = 0.05$, was used for all survey domain data analysis. **Table 7** displays the survey results of critical care NLRNs by survey period inclusive of P-value and sample size.

Progression Survey: satisfaction and commitment domain consists of questions focused on the NLRNs satisfaction of their job, work environment, and their intention to stay in their role. NLRNs who started in 2020 and 2021 had statistically significant decreases at all survey time periods in this domain compared with the benchmark of NLRNs starting in 2018. At the 12-month period, NLRNs in 2018 had a survey domain mean of 3.19 for the satisfaction and commitment domain, NLRNs in 2020 and 2021 had a decreased survey domain mean of 3.11 and 3.02, respectively. The Progression Survey: dissatisfaction domain consists of questions regarding the NLRNs dissatisfaction in the role, environment, and desire to find a new job in the next year. In comparison, this domain does not reflect the same trend as the progression satisfaction

Table 6
Critical care newly licensed registered nurses reasons for turnover insights

Turnover Reasons	2018 Critical Care NLRNs	2019 Critical Care NLRNs	2020 Critical Care NLRNs	2021 Critical Care NLRNS
NCLEX failure	0.54%	0.34%	0.84%	1.58%
Relocating out of area	20.4%	22.3%	19.8%	15.9%
Unsatisfactory performance	13.4%	12.5%	6%	7.2%
Obtained a position representing a different job experience	10.4%	13.8%	13.5%	15.9%
Left due to pandemic/crisis[a]	N/A	N/A	4%	0.8%
Travel nurse[b]	N/A	N/A	3.3%	3.8%

[a] Option added in 2020.
[b] Option added in 2021.

Table 7
Progression and CFGNES survey domains for newly licensed registered nurses in critical care areas by year and survey period

Survey Domain	Survey Time Period	2018 [Sample Size]	2019 (P Value) [Sample Size]	2020 (P Value) [Sample Size]	2021 (P Value) [Sample Size]
Progression Survey: Satisfaction and Commitment Domain	Initial	3.46 [4690]	3.46 (P=.74) [5490]	3.43ᵃ (P=.04) [5718]	3.35ᵃ (P<.001) [6922]
Progression Survey: Satisfaction and Commitment Domain	6-mo	3.23 [4109]	3.23 (P=.76) [4720]	3.19ᵃ (P<.001) [4947]	3.07ᵃ (P<.001) [5633]
Progression Survey: Satisfaction and Commitment Domain	12-mo	3.19 [3779]	3.2 (P=.28) [3831]	3.11ᵃ (P<.001) [4025]	3.02ᵃ (P<.001) [4449]
Progression Survey: Dissatisfaction Domain	Initial	1.67 [4690]	1.66 (P=.22) [5490]	1.66 (P=.10) [5718]	1.70ᵃ (P=.005) [6922]
Progression Survey: Dissatisfaction Domain	6-mo	1.87 [4109]	1.87 (P=.67) [4720]	1.87 (P=.74) [4947]	1.94ᵃ (P<.001) [5633]
Progression Survey: Dissatisfaction Domain	12-mo	1.93 [3779]	1.90ᵃ (P=.03) [3831]	1.94 (P=.75) [4025]	2.00ᵃ (P<.001) [4449]
Progression Survey: Competence	Initial	4.61 [4690]	4.64 (P=.74) [5490]	4.79ᵃ (P<.001) [5718]	4.83ᵃ (P<.001) [6922]
Progression Survey: Competence	6-mo	5.84 [4109]	5.85 (P=.63) [4720]	5.92ᵃ (P=.02) [4947]	6.01ᵃ (P<.001) [5633]
Progression Survey: Competence	12-mo	6.53 [3779]	6.55 (P=.82) [3831]	6.61ᵃ (P=.02) [4025]	6.69ᵃ (P<.001) [4449]
CFGNES: Patient Safety Domain	Initial	2.83 [4909]	2.82 (P=.77) [5622]	2.86ᵃ (P<.001) [5856]	2.83 (P=.69) [7054]
CFGNES: Patient Safety Domain	6-mo	3.03 [4208]	3.04 (P=.06) [4817]	3.04ᵃ (P=.04) [5048]	3.00ᵃ (P=.02) [5762]
CFGNES: Patient Safety Domain	12-mo	3.14 [3915]	3.15 (P=.52) [3948]	3.12 (P=.11) [4125]	3.08ᵃ (P<.001) [4594]
CFGNES: Support Domain	Initial	3.38 [4909]	3.39ᵃ (P=.02) [5622]	3.41ᵃ (P<.001) [5856]	3.38 (P=.96) [7054]
CFGNES: Support Domain	6-mo	3.33 [4208]	3.34 (P=.09) [4817]	3.34 (P=.13) [5048]	3.30ᵃ (P<.001) [5762]
CFGNES: Support Domain	12-mo	3.37 [3915]	3.39ᵃ (P=.04) [3948]	3.36 (P=.23) [4125]	3.33ᵃ (P<.001) [4594]

Statistical testing completed with the Mann–Whitney U test comparing to baseline year of 2018.
ᵃ Statistically significant α = 0.05.

and commitment domain in 2020. There were no statistically significant differences in 2020 NLRN survey data when compared with 2018 NLRN survey data. However, in 2021, there was statistically significant increase in the progression dissatisfaction domain, when compared with baseline, across all three survey periods. At the 12-month period in 2021, NLRNs survey domain mean was 2.00 compared with 1.93 in 2018.

To understand NLRNs self-assessment of competence, respondents were asked to "evaluate your progression in nursing competence". Using a whole number between the lowest point = 0 (novice) to the highest point = 10 (fully competent), where would you currently rate your nursing competence on this scale from 0 to 10. NLRNs in 2020 and 2021 reported statistically significant higher self-assessment mean of competence than NLRNs in 2018 across all three time periods (initial, 6 months, and 12 months). The NLRNs in 2020 and 2021 started with a higher self-assessment in competence (4.79 and 4.83, respectively) compared with 2018 (4.61) and at 12 months maintained a higher self-assessment in competence than 2018. However, 2018 NLRNs had a 41.65% increase in self-assessed competence from initial to 12-month surveys, whereas 2020 and 2021 NLRNs had a smaller increase (37.99% and 38.51%, respectively).

To further evaluate the experience of the NLRNs, the CFGNES support domain was analyzed. The CFGNES support domain consists of questions focused on how much the NLRN feels their coworkers, preceptors, and managers provide support and feedback. Across the years and survey time periods, there were varied results in survey data. There were statistically significant increases in the support domain for the initial survey in years 2019 (3.39) and 2020 (3.41) when compared with the 2018 initial benchmark (3.38). In addition, there was a statistically significant increase in 2019 at the 12-month time period compared with 2018. However, there was found to be statistically significant decreases in 2021 at 6 months (3.30) and 12 months (3.33) when compared with the same time in 2018 (initial 3.33 and 12 months 3.37).

To understand NLRNs assessment of care for their patients, CFGNES patient safety domain was selected. The CFGNES patient safety domain includes questions on organization, prioritization, and managing a patient assignment. There were no statistically significant differences in the year 2019 compared with the year 2018. For the years 2020 and 2021, there were varied results. Statistically significant increases in 2020 at the initial (2.86) and 6-month (3.04) survey period when compared with 2018 (initial 2.83, 6 months 3.03). However, in 2021, there was a reverse trend of statistically significant decreases in this domain at 6 months (3.00) and 12 months (3.08) when compared with 2018 (6 months 3.03, 12 months 3.14).

DISCUSSION

The COVID-19 pandemic has impacted NLRNs hired in critical care areas in many ways including increased numbers of NLRNs being hired directly into critical care areas, increased turnover rates, lower levels of NLRN satisfaction and commitment, varied results in readiness to practice and competency, and decreased feelings of support.

Increasing Hires in Critical Care Areas

From 2018 to 2022, there have been considerable increases in hiring NLRNs into critical care areas. Data trends differed by specialty area and if the area was considered adult or pediatric. Adult critical care units had large percentage increases in hires in 2020 to 2022. Pediatric critical care areas had slight increases in overall hires from

2019 to 2021 when compared with the 2018 benchmark. During the pandemic, higher numbers of adults were hospitalized for COVID-19 than pediatrics.[12] The increase in the patient population in the adult critical care units may have driven the hiring trends of organizations during these years. In 2022, the pediatric trend changed and there was an 83.14% increase in NLRNs hired into pediatric critical care units. Further investigation is needed to explore the increase in pediatric critical care NLRNs hires in 2022. Hiring data revealed pediatric critical care units had a larger percent increase in 2019 in hiring NLRNs than adult critical care units. In 2022, there were large percent increases in all the pediatric critical care units except the pediatric intermediate unit. The pediatric intermediate unit had negative percent growth in hires across 2020 to 2022.

Increase in Turnover Rates

As reported by Nursing Solutions Inc. (NSI), 105% of hospital workforce has turned over in the last 5 years.[16] For RNs specifically, turnover rates peaked in 2021 at 22.0%, and most recent data in 2022 reflect a rate of 19.9%.[16] NLRNs typically have higher turnover rates than registered nurses (RNs) who are more tenured.[16] However, organizations that have implemented NRP programs have shown a decrease in turnover of NLRNs.[11,17,18] During the pandemic, data from NLRNs who started in the critical care units participating in the Vizient/AACN NRP reflected similar trends as nationwide RNs, with increasing turnover over the years. Baseline turnover rate for critical care NLRNs in the Vizient/AACN NRP in 2018 was 10.13% and increased to 14.87% in 2021. Understanding why NLRNs are leaving is integral to sustaining, supporting, and reducing turnover. As reflected in the data, NLRNs leaving organizations due to "a job representing a different experience" increased by 5% from 2018 to 2021. In a study by Church and colleagues, 28.5% of NLRNs cited that they decided to leave their position due to pursuing career advancement and 27.3% listed having a lack of advancement opportunities as one of the reasons they were leaving their position.[17] Insights on what career advancement means to NLRNs and finding opportunities within the organizations to professionally grow can help organizations retain the organizational knowledge the NLRNs have gathered. This is crucial to understand for critical care NLRNs as organizations in this analysis have almost doubled the hiring numbers in the last 5 years.

Statistically Significant Difference in Satisfaction and Commitment

Ulrich and colleagues found that satisfaction with being an RN dropped from 62% in 2018 to 40% in 2021.[1] Data from the NLRNs hired into critical care in 2020 and 2021 showed a similar trend. There was a statistically significant decrease in the Progression Survey: satisfaction and commitment across all three time periods for NLRNs hired in 2020 (initial 3.43, 6 months 3.19, 12 months 3.11) and 2021 (initial 3.35, 6 months 3.07, 12 months 3.02) when comparing all years to the baseline of 2018 (initial 3.46, 6 months 3.23, 12 months 3.19). There are many factors that may have impacted the decrease in satisfaction and commitment in NLRNs in 2020 and 2021. Nursing students had significant impacts to their education which impacted their ability to practice skills and procedures and their self-assessed readiness to practice.[2] Graduates had delays in taking their NCLEX-RN examinations and took positions that were not their first choice due to changes in organizations.[4] NLRNs were faced with challenging nursing environments and reported anxiety related to uncertainty, concern for safety, vulnerability, changes in personal interactions and personal plans, abandonment from the health care team members and administration, and moral distress.[4,7,19,20] Although NLRNs reported these feelings, they still continued to report pride in their profession.[4,20] This is reflected in the NLRN survey data from 2020 and 2021. Although there are significant decreases in the domain means during these years, they still remain positive with scores above 3.0 on a 4.0 scale. Further research on survey data with this cohort of NLRNs can provide insights for academia and organizations on how to improve satisfaction and commitment in NLRNs. Furthermore, continued monitoring of NLRN satisfaction and commitment is needed in upcoming years as it is essential for the ongoing nursing workforce pipeline.

Varied Results in Readiness to Practice and Competency

In addition to satisfaction, understanding how the pandemic impacted critical care NLRNs in readiness to practice and competency will help support the future pipeline of RNs in the critical care area and provide insights for academia during pre-licensure preparation. When examining the number of critical care NLRNs who terminated due to NCLEX-RN failure, the percentage of turnovers only increased by 1% in 2021 when compared with the baseline in 2018. This is a minimal number of NLRNs, as it is only 1% of total turnovers in that year. NLRNs who started practice in 2020 and 2021 had their education impacted in various ways in response to the COVID-19 pandemic.[2-5] An increase in practice gaps for NLRNs starting in 2020 and 2021 has been found.[21] Of note, prevalent practice gaps were found in critical care, perinatal, and emergency NLRNs.[21]

However, when examining the Vizient/AACN NRP data, NLRNs in critical care self-reported statistically significant higher levels of competence in 2020 and 2021 when compared with baseline in 2018. To further understand this trend, the CFGNES patient safety domain was analyzed. Results showed statistically significant increases in the patient safety domain for NLRNs in initial (2.86) and 6-month (3.04) survey data for NLRNs who started in 2020 compared with 2018 (initial 2.83, 6 months 3.03). However, in 2021, the 6-month (3.00) and 12-month (3.08) patient safety survey domain had statistically significant decreases when comparing to 2018 NLRNs (6 months 3.03, 12 months 3.14). Owing to the size of the sample, these changes are statistically significantly but may lack a meaningful difference as there is minimal changes in the domain means that these results provide a mixed understanding of the preparedness with only a 1% change in NCLEX-RN turnover failures and statistically significant increase in self-reported competency levels of NLRNs entering the critical care areas. The increase in self-assessed competency may have been impacted by organization-specific pre-NRP courses aimed to address the skill gap that occurred due to decreased academic clinical rotations.[22] Of importance, the data examined were self-reported by NLRNs and do not include stakeholder assessments of preceptors or unit leaders which may provide additional insight to the level of competency of the NLRNs.

Statistically Significant Differences in Support

NLRNs in 2019 and 2020 reported statistically significant increases in the support domain compared with the baseline of 2018 for their initial surveys. In 2019, the initial survey support domain score was 3.39 and, in 2020, 3.41 compared with the baseline of 3.38 in 2018. In 2021, there was a statistically significant decrease in support reported at the 6-month (3.30) and 12-month (3.33) surveys compared with the 2018 baseline (6 months 3.33, 12 months 3.37). However, even though survey results were statistically significant, due to the small size of difference, they may not be meaningfully different.

The literature has shown that during COVID-19, strong unit leadership presence was found to provide a sense of safety and value to nurses, whereas macro-control and organizational support has been found to decrease health workers intention to leave.[10,23,24] Increasing macro-control can include providing education on emerging situations and providing safe working conditions.[23] Strong, clear managerial communication and interprofessional collaboration at an organization has been found to positively impact nurses' intention to stay in nursing.[24]

From a health care organizational perspective, support for NLRNs can come in many forms including NRPs. NRPs help to bridge the gap between academia and practice, provide the extra layer of support for NLRNs transitioning into nursing, and create a peer community and reducing turnover.[6,11,25] Approximately half of all hospitals in the United States have NRPs; although many differ in structure, all have similar goals including bolstering recruitment, increasing nursing and patient satisfaction, and reducing turnover.[26] The Institute of Medicine[27] report in 2010 recommended NRPs to assist NLRNs during their transition from academia to practice.

Over half of NLRNs cited that one of the reasons they stay in their first position is a sense of community among peers.[28] NLRNs reported that peer and manager support assisted them in navigating the pandemic.[7] NRPs offer a place in which NLRNs can meet each other, create a peer community, and relate to each other's experience. NRPs can support NLRNs and address opportunities that may arise due to emergent situations or gaps that academia and practice have identified. Organizations should have a plan in place for continuation of these programs during unforeseen events to provide the additional support and education that NLRNs need at this time.[4]

LIMITATIONS

Limitations of this program evaluation include that only member organizations in the national vendor NRP program were represented. NLRN data and hiring trends may not reflect the national landscape of NLRNs in critical care areas who are not part of the vendor program. In addition, NRP site coordinators were responsible for entering the NLRNs into the database. The national vendor program provides direction on definitions of each area; however, judgment of the NRP site coordinator is used for type of unit and turnover reasons. Last, all surveys that were completed for these organizations were used in the analysis. This could lead to a survivor bias, as 12-month survey data only represent NLRNs who did not turnover in their first year. It is also important to note that turnover data in this article reflect when NLRNs started their first day in the NRP and not hired into an organization. Last, initial surveys are completed typically on the NLRNs first day of NRP which varies between organizations.

SUMMARY

In conclusion, COVID-19 impacted the experiences of critical care NLRNs in both the adult and pediatric settings. Survey data from NRPs can help nurse leaders understand NLRNs self-assessed gaps, as well as trends in hiring and turnover, to assist organizations in individualizing strategies to better support and retain NLRNs. Health care organizations must continue to collaborate with academia to meet the needs of the clinical workforce in real time and help support the growing critical care NLRN population. Looking forward, 2022 hiring data can inform organizations of the current post-acute pandemic trends so that they can continue to plan and develop interventions to support the critical care workforce.

Health care organizations must reflect on lessons learned during the COVID-19 pandemic. Emergent situations will continue to occur and findings from research on how to support health care workers can help inform organizational best practices including operationalizing and sustaining NRPs.

This information contained in this article was based in part on the Vizient/AACN Nurse Residency Program maintained by the Vizient/AACN.

CLINICS CARE POINTS

- Data revealed an increase in hiring and turnovers of critical care newly licensed registered nurses (NLRNs) during the pandemic.
- Engagement and support for NLRNs during their first year of nursing practice is key.
- Nurse Residency Program can improve retention for NLRNs and bridge the academia-practice gap.
- Reflecting on pandemic lessons learned while engaging critical care NLRNs and academic partners can assist in planning for future unplanned events.

DISCLOSURE

A. Renkema was previously employed by Vizient, Inc and K. Gallagher is currently employed at Vizient, Inc.

REFERENCES

1. Ulrich B, Cassidy L, Barden C, et al. National nurse work environments - October 2021: a status report. Crit Care Nurse 2022;42(5):58–70.
2. Musallam E, Flinders B A. Senior BSN students' confidence, comfort, and perception of readiness for clinical practice: the impacts of COVID-19. Int J Nurs Educ Scholarsh 2021;18(1):20200097.
3. Martin B, Kaminski-Ozturk N, Smiley R, et al. Assessing the impact of the COVID-19 pandemic on nursing education: a national study of prelicensure RN programs. Journal of Nursing Regulation 2023;14(1):S1–67.
4. Crismon D, Mansfield KJ, Hiatt SO, et al. COVID-19 pandemic impact on experiences and perceptions of nurse graduates. J Prof Nurs 2021;37(5):857–65.
5. Smith SM, Buckner M, Jessee MA, et al. Impact of COVID-19 on new graduate nurses' transition to practice: loss or gain? Nurse Educ 2021;46(4):209–14.
6. Casey K, Oja KJ, Makic MBF. The lived experiences of graduate nurses transitioning to professional practice during a pandemic. Nurs Outlook 2021;69(6):1072–80.
7. Sessions LC, Ogle KT, Lashley M, et al. Coming of age during coronavirus: new nurses' perceptions of transitioning to practice during a pandemic. J Cont Educ Nurs 2021;52(6):294–300.
8. Djukic M, Padhye N, Ke Z, et al. Associations between the COVID-19 pandemic and new nurses' transition to practice outcomes: a multi-site, longitudinal study. Journal of Nursing Regulation 2023;14(1):42–9.
9. Gordon JM, Magbee T, Yoder LH. The experiences of critical care nurses caring for patients with COVID-19 during the 2020 pandemic: a qualitative study. Appl Nurs Res 2021;59:151418.
10. Brockopp D, Monroe M, Davies CC, et al. COVID-19: the lived experience of critical care nurses. J Nurs Adm 2021;51(7/8):374–8.
11. Goode CJ, Lynn MR, McElroy D, et al. Lessons learned from 10 years of research on a post-baccalaureate nurse residency program. J Nurs Adm 2013;43(2):73–9.

12. Couture A, Iuliano AD, Chang HH, et al. Estimating COVID-19 hospitalizations in the United States with surveillance data using a Bayesian hierarchical model: modeling study. JMIR Public Health Surveill 2022;8(6):e34296.
13. Vizient/AACN Nurse Residency ProgramTM. Irving, TX: Vizient, Inc. Accessed 1 September, 2023. https://www.vizientinc.com/what-we-do/operations-and-quality/vizient-aacn-nurse-residency-program.
14. Casey K, Fink RR, Krugman AM, et al. The graduate nurse experience. J Nurs Adm: J Nurs Adm 2004;34(6):303–11.
15. Casey, K., & Fink, R. Psychometrics Casey Fink Graduate Nurse Experience Survey 2006. Accessed August 3, 2023. https://www.caseyfinksurveys.com/graduate-nurse-experience-survey-2006.
16. NSI National Health Care Retention & RN Staffing Report, 2023. Accessed 1 September, 2023. https://www.nsinursingsolutions.com/Documents/Library/NSI_National_Health_Care_Retention_Report.pdf.
17. Cadmus E, Roberts ML. First year outcomes: program evaluation of a statewide nurse residency program. J Nurs Adm 2022;52(12):672–8.
18. Ulrich B, Krozek C, Early S, et al. Improving retention, confidence, and competence of new graduate nurses: results from a 10-year longitudinal database. Nurs Econ 2010;28(6):363–76.
19. Bongiorno AW, Armstrong N, Moore GA, et al. Impressions of the nursing profession among nursing students and new graduates during the first wave of COVID-19: a qualitative content analysis. Nurse Educ 2023;48(4):204–8.
20. Mannino JE, Watters P, Cotter E, et al. The future capacity of the nursing workforce: COVID-19 pandemic's impacts on new nurses and nursing students toward the profession. Nurse Educ 2021;46(6):342–8.
21. Grubaugh M, Africa L, Mallory C. Where do we go from here? Nurse Leader 2022; 20(2):134–40.
22. Warren JI, Zipp JS, Goodwin J, et al. Overcoming the disruption of clinical nursing education: a statewide hospital-academic initiative. J Nurses Prof Dev 2022;38(4):253–6.
23. Çetin Aslan E, Türkmen İ, Top M. The effect of macro-control and organizational support perception on nurses and physicians intention to quit during the COVID-19 pandemic. J Nurs Scholarsh 2023;55(4):843–52.
24. Yu G, Kovner CT, Glassman K, et al. The impact of the early COVID-19 pandemic on registered nurses' intent to stay in nursing. Pol Polit Nurs Pract 2023;24(3): 168–77.
25. Alsalamah YS, Al Hosis K, Al Harbi A, et al. Student to nurse transition and the nurse residency program: a qualitative study of new graduate perceptions. J Prof Nurs 2022;42:195–200.
26. Sutor Amy, et al. Nurse residency programs: providing organizational value. Delaware journal of public health 2020;6(1):58–61.
27. Institute of Medicine. The future of nursing: leading change, advancing health. Washington, DC: The National Academies Press; 2011.
28. Church CD, Schalles R, Wise T. The newly-licensed registered nurse workforce: looking back to move forward. Nurs Outlook 2023;71(1):101904.

Supporting and Retaining Nurses in Trying Times

M. Dave Hanson, MSN, RN, ACNS-BC, NEA-BC[a,†],
Marian Altman, PhD, RN, CNS-BC, CCRN[b],
Susan Lacey, PhD, RN, CNL, FAAN[c,*]

KEYWORDS

- Nurse retention • Strategies to improve nurse retention • Recognition • COVID-19
- Leadership

KEY POINTS

- Nurses have experienced unprecedented times during the coronavirus disease 2019 pandemic.
- Rebuilding trust should be a key leadership strategy in today's health-care system.
- Leaders should leverage meaningful recognition programs to provide a sense of belonging.

INTRODUCTION

The nursing profession has witnessed its share of challenging and trying times including toxic or unhealthy work environments, unsustainable workloads, an aging workforce, inadequate staffing, nurse burnout, staff retention, inadequately trained staff, and an increase in workplace violence. However, the biggest issue the nursing profession has faced began in March 2020 when New York City became the epicenter of the coronavirus disease 2019 (COVID-19) outbreak in the United States.[1] The novel coronavirus pandemic has forever changed the face of the nursing profession, and some would argue the profession still has not fully recovered. In fact, the pandemic only exacerbated the problems and challenges the profession was experiencing. Nurses were left demoralized, burned out, overwhelmed, and sadly many simply left the profession altogether.

The purpose of this article is to describe some of the issues brought on by the pandemic but to, even more importantly, offer solutions and innovative strategies

a Society of Critical Care Medicine, 2050 North Clark Street #301, Chicago, IL 60614, USA;
b American Association of Critical-Care Nurses, 416 River Bluff Lane, King & Queen Courthouse, VA 23085, USA; c Society of Critical Care Medicine, 2900 Grouse Lane, Rolling Meadows, IL 60008, USA
† Deceased
* Corresponding author.
E-mail address: slacey@sccm.org

Crit Care Nurs Clin N Am 36 (2024) 353–365
https://doi.org/10.1016/j.cnc.2024.01.007
0899-5885/24/© 2024 Elsevier Inc. All rights reserved.

ccnursing.theclinics.com

on how to support and retain nurses in trying times. We as a profession must be better prepared for the next challenge—big or small—that comes our way. No one is better prepared to resolve the barriers our profession faces than nurses themselves. Solutions should include being prepared with tools and resources to allow us to thrive and survive during the day-to-day experiences in health care as well as in unprecedented times such as another pandemic.

SIGNIFICANCE OF RETAINING NURSES

According to the American Association of Colleges of Nursing, nursing is the nation's largest health-care profession, with nearly 5.2 million registered nurses (RNs) nationwide. Of all licensed RNs, 89% are employed in nursing.[2] Yet, there remains a critical shortage of RNs to safely care for patients and their family members. Why is nurse retention such an important issue to tackle? It is simple. It is the key to creating safe passage through the health-care system.

It is been said that nurses are the glue that holds the health-care system together. Another way of looking at it would be if you were to remove nurses from health care, then the very system of health care as we know it would cease to function. In other words, patients and their families would be at great risk of harm and injury because nurses, the very architects of quality and safety would be missing from the health-care system in which consumers have come to rely on. Having and retaining a competent and qualified nursing profession is in everyone's best interest.

The public counts on nurses to be there in good and bad times. Nurses continue to garner the most trusted rating from Americans among a diverse list of professions, a distinction they have held for more than 2 decades according to the 2023 Gallup survey.[3] Retaining nurses is key to many things including enhanced clinical outcomes, improved patient satisfaction, better nursing satisfaction, and a safely functioning health-care system.[4]

HISTORY OF THE COVID-19 PANDEMIC AND ITS IMPACT ON THE NURSING PROFESSION

COVID-19 caused an onslaught of patients on an unprepared health-care system.[5] No one was prepared for how sick these patients would be and how quickly the virus would spread. Not only were health-care workers unsure of how to manage the clinical course but also the lack of critical supplies such as personal protection equipment (PPE) and even ventilators led to profound complexity of patient management.[6] The lack of PPE left health-care workers vulnerable to catching the virus while losing trust in their leadership for failing to protect them. The lack of ventilators meant rationing this lifesaving equipment causing health-care workers to triage their patients to determine who would get them causing many ethical dilemmas. This need to triage patients due to scarce resource at this scale had not been experienced by the majority of health-care personnel during the course of their professional lives.[7]

Due to the moratorium on visitation, families were left to wonder how their loved ones were doing and nurses were at the sharp end of this communication, which would primarily be managed by phone calls. In some cases, nurses began the innovative approach of using FaceTime or computer tablets to help their patients communicate with family members unless they were unable to do so, given the severity of their condition.[8] For many, families were told their loved one died without the love and care most often provided during these times. This added additional stress and strain on the nurses caring for the dying and comforting the families as best they could from afar.

Not only were there patient crises and ethical dilemmas but also colleagues of health-care workers were also dying from COVID-19. From January 1, 2020, to October 12, 2021, the Centers for Disease and Control reported 440,044 cases among health-care workers and 1469 deaths, which was higher than the general population.[9]

STRATEGIES FOR RETAINING NURSES IN THE POSTPANDEMIC ERA

During the pandemic trust eroded between hospital leadership and nurses due to lack of PPE and poor staffing. These issues were coupled with hiring travelers at rates full-time employees would never receive. Nurse leaders also were faced with identifying meaningful strategies for supporting frontline nurses who were both physically and emotionally exhausted. Leadership would rely on these strategies while alienating their regular staff. What can be done about issues mitigating the lack of trust nurses have for hospital leadership? **Table 1** lists issues at play and reasonable strategies for retaining nurses.[10] Trust, staffing, compensation, and mental health are all essential elements for an engaged nursing workforce. Leadership can easily put these concepts into action by walking-the walk and talking-the talk. In other words, leaders must always be authentic in their words and actions.

Trust

The concept of trust is paramount between staff and their leaders. Trust is the glue that sustains the relationship. Rose Sherman's article in "My American Nurse," citing work from David Horsanger, identified 8 pillars of trust successful leaders possess found in **Table 2**.[11] These attributes provide staff with the necessary belief and trust in their leaders to stay in their positions.

Staffing

Staffing should be flexible and not fixed or predetermined, given the conditions of the patients on the unit at any given time. Leaders should use flexible staffing at peak times, particularly during admissions and discharges. Leaders should also seek additional staffing if the collective acuity is considerably higher than usual. Failure to do so puts nurses and patients at risk for harm.[12]

Compensation

Traditional approaches to staffing challenges such as sign-on bonuses and use of traveler or temporary staff provide temporary relief; however, such measures often compound long-term staffing challenges and carry additional unintended negative consequences.[13] Instead of these options, leadership should look at ways to

Table 1 Issues and strategies for retaining nurses[10]	
Issue	**Strategy**
Trust	Rebuild trust by listening to what nurses have to say about their work experiences and following through
Staffing	Staffing levels should be safe to avoid burnout and adverse clinical outcomes. Staff for peak times around discharges and admissions
Compensation	Do not treat nurses as commodities. Replace sign-on bonuses with retention bonuses
Value mental health	Provide access to online or virtual individual and/or group mental health providers

Table 2	
Eight pillars of trust with definitions[11]	
Pillar	**Definition**
Clarity	People trust clarity not ambiguous statements and behavior
Compassion	Caring beyond oneself
Character	Doing what is right vs what is easy
Competency	Demonstrating capability and relevance
Commitment	Standing with staff through difficult times
Connection	Maintaining rituals around comradery
Contribution	Seeking quick wins. People respond to results
Consistency	Implementing routine behaviors that benefit staff

compensate regular staff at higher rates during these peak times. Premium pay for regular staff can be used to recognize and support staff while also fostering appropriate staffing and not just paying staff more money to work short staffed. It is demoralizing to know someone with no experience on a unit is getting premium pay when regular staff are not. This can breed resentment, not just for the new staff but administration in general.

Access to Mental Health Services

A study published in 2021 that reviewed mental health outcomes for nurses in 25 studies found that 32% experienced anxiety, 40.6% experienced stress, 32% experienced depression, 18.6% reported post traumatic stress disorder (PTSD), and 38.3% experienced insomnia signaling significant risk factors for mental health issues while caring for COVID-19 patients.[14] The significance of this study underscores the importance of good mental health in the nursing workforce and its impact on clinical outcomes and nurse well-being.

This means during times of real or perceived crisis, leaders should consider mental health support.[15] This could come in the form of access to individual or group sessions with mental health professionals or virtual visits. Staff should be encouraged to ask for this assistance and told that doing so is not a sign of weakness but of strength.

Nurse Empowerment and Autonomy

Nurse empowerment has long been a source of discussion specifically related to the mostly all women profession of nursing. There is a long history of gender, voice, and autonomy being always at a crossroads in our hierarchical health-care facilities. Despite advancements, we still live in the power differentials that exist in our workplace. Lateral violence, bullying, and incivility can be considered side effects of these historical issues, which can be related to gender oppression.[16] Empowerment has often been put into the perspective of psychological empowerment, which refers to how the individual's motivation in their workplace is impacted by workplace structures. Higher levels of psychological empowerment have been linked to improved job satisfaction and lower levels of burnout.[17]

A similar concept, autonomy, can also be explored within the context of our complex health-care systems. Autonomy is the ability to act freely without inhibitions. Nurse managers and other leaders have the ultimate capability and capacity to create conditions to encourage nurses to use their autonomy based on their expertise.[18] Creating the right conditions for improving autonomy and empowerment needs an authentic and transformational leader as opposed to a transactional leader. Involving frontline nurses in decisions that influence their practice is a top strategy. Recognizing each nurse for their unique perspectives and talents can lead to feelings of inclusion and belonging that supports nurse confidence and empowerment.

Healthy Work Environments

The need to retain nurses in the workforce continues to be an issue in the post-COVID-19 pandemic era. Focusing on creating a healthy work environment (HWE) has been shown as one method to address turnover.[19] In 2005, the American Association of Critical-Care Nurses (AACN) issued the *AACN Standards for Establishing and Sustaining Healthy Work Environments: A Journey to Excellence*[20] to actively promote an HWE to support and foster patient care. Six standards were identified that must be in place to create and ensure an HWE. The standards are as follows: skilled communication, true collaboration, effective decision-making, appropriate staffing, meaningful recognition, and authentic leadership. All six standards are interconnected and considered essential. The HWE standards align with the core competencies for health-care professions recommended by the National Academy of Medicine and with the American Nurses' Association *Code of Ethics for Nurses*. The standards represent evidence-based and relationship-centered principles for professional performance.

There are many valid and reliable research studies conducted around the world spanning 2 decades that support the tenets of the HWE standards and highlight the need to focus on creating an HWE to achieve both positive patient and nurse outcomes.[21–29] See **Table 3**.

Despite the long-standing evidence supporting the link between HWE and positive outcomes, a 2021 survey[30] showed that the health of nurse work environments has declined dramatically since a previous 2018 study.[31] Therefore, action is urgently needed to create an HWE to support and retain nurses. One of the AACN HWE Standards is Meaningful Recognition.[20] There is a myriad of literature about recognition, specifically what recognition activities are the most meaningful to the individual. Therefore, the focus of this article will be on the HWE standard of meaningful recognition because it relates to recruiting, retaining, and supporting nurses in trying times.

Peer-to-peer recognition

Peer-to-peer recognition occurs when one colleague recognizes or acknowledges another colleague for their skill, something they did, or their talent. This is a powerful form of recognition because it is from a peer who shares and understands the unique day-to-day challenges of the job. Peer-to-peer recognition enhances the unit culture, fosters inclusion, strengthens team morale, and increases employee engagement.[32]

Table 3
Healthy work environment outcomes table

Patients Cared for in HWEs	Nurses Who Work in HWEs
• Experience less mortality and failure to be rescued[21] • Have better survival rates from in-hospital cardiac arrest[21] • Encounter fewer hospital-acquired conditions and adverse events[22] • Encounter fewer readmissions[23] • Report better overall quality of care[24]	• Report increased job satisfaction[26] • Report lower levels of burnout and compassion fatigue[27] • Are more likely to stay in their current job[28] • Report less staff turnover[28] • Decreased nurse turnover rates[29]

Examples of peer-to-peer recognition include the following: a board where employees post their recognitions on the unit, a software program where employees submit their recognitions, or shout outs during unit meetings or on social media. Some peer-to-peer recognition programs use a point-based system that can be used to select a gift, monetary recognition, free lunch, or coffee at the organization. Other programs provide the employee with certificates and awards.

Patient to nurse recognition

Many patients and families recognize nurses or the unit where they are being cared for by writing a thank you note, sending food, or making a donation in the unit or nurses' honor. Another example of a patient to nurse recognition program is the DAISY Award for Extraordinary Nurses.[33] The DAISY Foundation was formed in 1999 by a family deeply affected by the care provided by a nurse to their family member to honor and celebrate the special things that nurses do every day while caring for their patients. Patients may share their stories and thanks by nominating a nurse for a DAISY Award. A committee of nurses reviews the nominations to determine which nurses receive the DAISY Awards.

Unit excellence awards recognition

Another form of meaningful recognition is unit excellence awards. There are many examples of unit excellence awards. Many are obtained through nursing professional organizations. The AACN Beacon Award for Excellence is an award that recognizes the nation's top hospital units.[34] The award signifies exceptional care through improved outcomes and greater overall satisfaction. A Beacon unit has a positive and supportive work environment often with greater collaboration between colleagues and leaders, higher morale and lower turnover. The award recognizes units who have a consistent and systematic approach to evidence-based care and outcomes. The bronze, silver, and gold award levels signify achievement and progression on the journey to excellence.

The Emergency Nurses Association Lantern Award is granted to emergency departments that demonstrate exceptional and innovative performance because it relates to leadership, practice, education, advocacy, or research.[35,36] Successful applicants demonstrate a variety of diverse initiatives with quantifiable outcomes, sustained improvements, and innovative processes.

The Academy of Medical-Surgical Nurses sponsors the PRISM Award to provide special recognition to the exemplary practice of medical-surgical units. PRISM stands for Premier Recognition In the Specialty of Med-surg. The PRISM award recognizes units that achieve sustained excellence in patient/care management, holistic patient care, elements of interprofessional care, professional concept, and nursing teamwork and collaboration.

Organizational recognition programs

An organization recognition program for employees is a key component of a healthy workplace. Although recognition, which is tied to what we do and not who we are, is important, perhaps the focus should be on valuing. Value is about appreciating the worth of someone for who they are and for their unique contribution to the workplace.[37] The act of valuing another just may be the driver of engagement more than recognition. Programs dedicated to showing that employees are valued may be on track to improve employee engagement[38] and may result in higher levels of loyalty, productivity, and profit.[39] Value actions include a frank and honest discussion of what value means to individuals and groups—your department, your workgroup. When giving feedback, focus on the value others bring to the team, their unique contributions. The link to belonging is clear. If one feels valued, we believe they would feel like they belonged to the team and feel celebrated as a valuable team member.

Other formal organizational recognition programs may include recognition strategies to include formal recognition in front of peers, handwritten notes, length of service awards, awards for special accomplishments such as certifications, academic achievements or publications and nominations for awards both within and external to the organization.

One of the most widely recognized formal organizational level recognition programs is the Magnet Recognition Program. This program was developed in 1990 by the American Nurses Credentialing Center to recognize health-care organizations that provide nursing excellence and to disseminate successful nursing practices and strategies.[40] It is the premier international acknowledgment of nursing excellence in health-care organizations. The program was formed in response to the findings of a 1983 study conducted by the American Academy of Nursing's Task Force on Nursing Practice. The Magnet Recognition Program focuses on advancing 3 goals within each organization.

1. Promoting quality in a setting that supports professional practice.
2. Identifying excellence in the delivery of nursing services to patients.
3. Disseminating best practices in nursing services.

The Magnet Model is made up of 5 key components that focus on measuring quality, patient care, and performance outcomes. These are as follows: transformational leadership, structural empowerment, exemplary professional practice, new knowledge, innovation and improvement, and empirical quality results. See **Table 4** for more information.

There is much research surrounding the positive outcomes associated with Magnet designation. Studies show that job satisfaction and employee retention rates are higher, there are positive impact on patient safety, decreased lengths of stays, and fewer adverse patient events.[41]

Nurse Engagement

Today's health-care environment brings sharp focus on the need to ensure nurses are engaged and committed to their work. Nurse engagement is used to describe a nurse's

Table 4 Forces of magnetism	
Force of Magnetism	**Definition**
Transformational leadership	The ability to adjust to changing demands within the health-care industry by updating an organization's behaviors, values, and processes when necessary
Structural empowerment	Nurses in a facility can contribute to establishing the standards and processes they use at work
Exemplary professional practice	Nursing practice ensures each patient receives the care they need
New knowledge, innovation, and improvement	Organizations use evidence-based practices and research when implementing clinical and operational processes and to focus on generating innovation in the health-care field
Empirical quality results	Focuses on determining how solid processes and structures can positively impact the nursing staff, the entire organization and the care systems

satisfaction with their jobs and their commitment to the unit, the organization and the nursing profession. Highly engaged teams have better retention rates, higher patient satisfaction, improved patient outcomes, and improved organizational performance. Research has shown that nurse engagement scores correlate directly with safety, quality, and patient outcomes.[42]

Drivers of Engagement

Organizations with high engagement demonstrate that their employees are valued. Employees feel recognized and rewarded for their work. Authors Dempsey and Assi best articulate the balance necessary to achieving an engaged workforce in the following insightful quote. "To attain and maintain an engaged nursing workforce, leaders must ensure that the inherent rewards of the job—saving lives, helping families, important work—and the added rewards of compensation, privileges, and benefits outweigh the inherent stresses of the job that result from its complexity, the sense of responsibility, scheduling and productivity requirements, and, sometimes, dysfunctional systems."[43] Other drivers of engagement are listed in **Table 5**.

Nurse leaders profoundly influence employee engagement.[43] Leadership sets the engagement tone of the unit with their words and actions. Anecdotally, when nurses see their leaders engaged, they are more likely to be engaged themselves. Strategies that nurse leaders may use to reengage staff include the following: reconnecting staff with their purpose, creating an environment with psychological safety, reinvigorating share governance, providing meaningful recognition regularly, and offering professional development opportunities. A culture of engagement can also be cultivated by hiring the appropriate talent that are committed to the mission, vision, and values of the unit and the organization.

Measures of Nurse Engagement

Health systems typically track staff engagement through assessments such as the Gallup Employee Engagement Survey, the Glint Survey, or Press Ganey Workforce Engagement Solutions. Press Ganey is a provider of patient experience measurement, performance analytics, and strategic advisory solutions for health-care organizations. Press Ganey measures nurse engagement through proprietary survey instruments

Table 5 Drivers of nurse engagement	
Autonomy	**Nurses Are Trusted to Make Appropriate Decisions**
Positive relationships with a strong support network and mutual respect within the team	Relationships built on true collaboration and mutual respect
Opportunities for professional development	Consistent feedback, continuing education furthering their education, mentorship programs where experienced staff partner with newer staff to provide support and guidance
Effective communication that is open and frequent	Health-care team members are as proficient in their communication skills because they are in their clinical skills
Authentic leaders who promote and role model nursing leadership	Leaders that fully embrace a HWE, authentically live it and engage others
Purpose and meaning in work	Connecting your purpose or the what you do to the why you do it and the opportunity to use your knowledge and strengths

designed to assess multiple facets of the nurse experience, including nurse engagement, nurse job satisfaction, and the nurse work environment. This includes the Press Ganey National Database of Nursing Quality Indicators measuring nurse satisfaction, practice environment, and nurse-sensitive measures. Measures of nurse engagement include autonomy, professional development, leadership access and responsiveness, interprofessional relationships, quality of nursing care, resources and staffing, and nurse-to-nurse teamwork and collaboration. Tracking this data is so important for the realization of an HWE and is often required for many of the organizational and/ or unit recognitions previously referenced.

Disengagement

In the postpandemic world, many staff are disengaged from their work. Disengagement can be caused by internal or external factors. Examples of internal factors are feeling a lack of purpose or meaning in the work. For some nurses, disengagement is a result of multiple COVID-19 pandemic surges. Multiple COVID-19 pandemic surges can leave nurses even more burnt-out, disheartened, overwhelmed, and disengaged. Another cause of disengagement is lack of meaningful recognition and lack of professional development opportunities. Examples include poor communication within an organization, lack of resources such as staffing to provide safe and effective care, and lack of or limited equipment needed to provide care.[44] Focusing on nurse engagement strategies that support, value, and empower nurses is essential to reengaging staff, creating an HWE, improving patient outcomes, and supporting and retaining nurses.

Shared Governance

Another method to support and retain nurses and a driver of engagement is to implement shared governance. Shared governance is a nursing practice model that was first introduced more than 4 decades ago that empowers and engages the front-line nurse in decision-making process and goals of an organization shifting decision-making from a top–down approach to a more collaborative approach. As suggested by O'Grady and Clavelle, the nursing profession should move from shared governance to professional governance.[45] Professional governance is foundational to nurse empowerment. The main principles of this form of governance include ownership, shared accountability, empowerment, team building, collaborative partnerships, leadership, innovation, autonomy, and practice equity.[46] Organizations with professional or shared governance structures move from a hierarchical structure to a councilor structure to ensure that the nurses are involved in the governance of professional issues, have their voices heard, and have an opportunity to impact outcomes through a formal structure such as a unit nursing council with a charter that identifies roles and responsibilities of both members and organizational leaders.[44]

Implementing shared governance is associated with improved nurse-sensitive indicators and improved job satisfaction through engaging direct care nurses in policy development, and revisions.[47] Shared governance is also a strategy for internal succession planning by assisting nurses to develop their leadership skills.

According to Porter-O'Grady, "Now more accurately identified as professional governance, shared governance focuses on the creation of a structural framework for nursing practice consistent with the frameworks that govern other major professions."[48] However, implementing professional governance can be challenging. Frontline nurse buy-in and participation may be difficult to obtain due to the increased workload and the time commitment associated with professional governance. Nurses are balancing their work commitment with personal responsibilities, and some are also pursuing advanced degrees. It is essential that nightshift and nurses who only work weekends are involved in professional governance. Some organizations offer governance council meetings at night or on weekends regularly. It is also essential that nurse leaders provide education about the governance process and include direct care nurses in the creation of the model to instill trust and assist with buy-in.[49]

SUMMARY

Since the days of Florence Nightingale during the Crimean War, both individual nurses and the profession as a whole have witnessed challenging and trying times. The COVID-19 pandemic brought with it unique circumstances that strained the very health-care systems in which nurses work. However, our profession is resilient, and we have learned to navigate the pitfalls that would have upended many other professions. The key lesson we have learned is that supporting and retaining nurses in challenging and trying times are essential to our longevity as a profession.

CLINICS CARE POINTS

- Two of the most important contributors to nurse retention are meaningful recognition and nurse autonomy and decision-making.
- Employee recognition programs should acknowledge reward and achievement.
- Meaningful recognition boosts morale and motivation and is associated with improved job satisfaction and organizational outcomes.
- Nurses empowered to participate in decision-making are more engaged and provide higher quality patient care.

ACKNOWLEDGMENTS

The authors would like to acknowledge Dr Caryl Goodyear, PhD, RN, NEA-BC, FAAN for her wisdom, guidance, and assistance with this article.

DISCLOSURE

The authors have no monetary or other types of conflicts of interest to disclose regarding this article.

REFERENCES

1. Holshue ML, DeBolt C, Lindquist S, et al. First case of 2019 novel coronavirus in the United States. N Engl J Med 2020 Mar 5;382(10):929–36.
2. Smiley RA, Allgeyer RL, Shobo Y, et al. The 2022 national nursing workforce survey. J Nurs Regul 2023 Apr;14(1):S1–90.
3. Brenan M. Nurses retain top ethics rating in the U.S., but below 2020 high. In: Gallup. 2023 Jan 10. Available at: https://news.gallup.com/poll/467804/nurses-retain-top-ethics-rating-below-2020-high.aspx. Accessed July 30, 2023.
4. Flynn, R. The impact of nurse retention on patient care and outcomes: a closer look. In: StaffGarden. 2023 Aug 8. Available at: https://www.staffgarden.com/insight-detail/the-impact-of-nurse-retention. Accessed July 30, 2023.
5. Turale S, Meechamnan C, Kunaviktikul W. Challenging times: ethics, nursing and the COVID-19 pandemic. Int Nurs Rev 2020;67(2):164–7.

6. Zhao Z, Li R, Ma Y, et al. Supporting technologies for COVID-19 prevention: systemized review. JMIRx Med 2022;3(2):e30344.
7. Gristina GR, Piccinni M. COVID-19 pandemic in ICU. Limited resources for many patients: approaches and criteria for triaging. Minerva Anestesiol 2021;87(12): 1367–79. https://doi.org/10.23736/S0375-9393.21.15736-0.
8. Bloom-Feshbach K, Bullington BW, Wahid N, et al. Using digital tablets to humanize patient care during the COVID-19 pandemic. Acad Med 2021;96(2):e9–10. https://doi.org/10.1097/ACM.0000000000003792.
9. Lin S, Deng X, Ryan I, et al. COVID-19 symptoms and deaths among healthcare workers, United States. Emerg Infect Dis 2022;28(8):1624–41. https://doi.org/10.3201/eid2808.212200.
10. Jorgenson, S. E. (2018). Nurses Aren't Commodities. www.KevinMD.com.
11. Horsager D. The trust edge. New York, NY: Simon and Schuster; 2012.
12. Butler M, Schultz TJ, Halligan P, et al. Hospital nurse-staffing models and patient- and staff-related outcomes. Cochrane Database Syst Rev 2011. https://doi.org/10.1002/14651858.CD007019.pub2.
13. Hospital Careers. Top 12 hospitals paying nursing bonuses. June 1, 2022 at https://hospitalcareers.com/blog/hospitals-paying-nurse-bonuses/. Accessed July 30, 2023.
14. Varghese A, George G, Kondaguli SV, et al. Decline in the mental health of nurses across the globe during COVID-19: a systematic review and meta-analysis. J Glob Health 2021;11:05009.
15. Riedel B, Horen SR, Reynolds A, et al. Mental health disorders in nurses during the COVID-19 pandemic: implications and coping strategies. Front Public Health 2021;9:707358.
16. Woodward KF. Individual nurse empowerment: a concept analysis. Nurs Forum 2020;55(2):136–43.
17. Orlowska, A., Laguna, M. Structural and psychological empowerment in explaining job satisfaction and burnout in nurses: A two-level investigation. 2023; JNM Article ID 9958842 10.1155/2023/9958842.
18. Gottlieb LN, Gottlieb B, Bitzas V. Creating empowering conditions for nurses with workplace autonomy and agency: how healthcare leaders could be guided by strengths-based nursing and healthcare leadership (SBNH-L). J Healthc Leader 2021;13:169–81.
19. Sweeney CD, Wiseman R. Retaining the best: recognizing what meaningful recognition is to nurses as a strategy for nurse leaders. J Nurs Adm 2023; 53(2):81–7. https://doi.org/10.1097/NNA.0000000000001248.
20. American Association of Critical Care Nurses. AACN Standards for Establishing and Sustaining Healthy Work Environments: A Journey to Excellence, 2nd edition, 2016.
21. Olds DM, Aiken LH, Cimiotti JP, et al. Association of nurse work environment and safety climate on patient mortality: a cross-sectional study. Int J Nurs Stud 2017; 74:155–61. https://doi.org/10.1016/j.ijnurstu.2017.06.004.
22. Kelly D, Kutney-Lee A, Lake ET, et al. The critical care work environment and nurse-reported health care-associated infections. Am J Crit Care 2013;22(6): 482–8. https://doi.org/10.4037/ajcc2013298.
23. Ma C, McHugh MD, Aiken LH. Organization of hospital nursing and 30-day readmissions in medicare patients undergoing surgery. Med Care 2015;53(1):65–70. https://doi.org/10.1097/MLR.0000000000000258.
24. Gensimore MM, Maduro RS, Morgan MK, et al. The effect of nurse practice environment on retention and quality of care via burnout, work characteristics, and

resilience: a moderated mediation model. J Nurs Adm 2020;50(10):546–53. https://doi.org/10.1097/NNA.0000000000000932.

26. Al Sabei SD, Labrague LJ, Miner Ross A, et al. Nursing work environment, turn-over intention, job burnout, and quality of care: the moderating role of job satis-faction. J Nurs Scholarsh 2020;52(1):95–104. https://doi.org/10.1111/jnu.12528.

27. Nantsupawat A, Kunaviktikul W, Nantsupawat R, et al. Effects of nurse work envi-ronment on job dissatisfaction, burnout, intention to leave. Int Nurs Rev 2017; 64(1):91–8. https://doi.org/10.1111/inr.12342.

28. Labrague LJ, Al Sabei S, Al Rawajfah O, et al. Authentic leadership and nurses' motivation to engage in leadership roles: the mediating effects of nurse work environment and leadership self-efficacy. J Nurs Manag 2021;29(8):2444–52. https://doi.org/10.1111/jonm.13448.

29. Al Yahyaei A, Hewison A, Efstathiou N, et al. Nurses' intention to stay in the work environment in acute healthcare: a systematic review. J Res Nurs 2022;27(4): 374–97. https://doi.org/10.1177/17449871221080731.

30. Ulrich B, Cassidy L, Barden C, et al. National nurse work environments - october 2021: a status report. Crit Care Nurse 2022;42:5.

31. Ulrich B, Barden C, Cassidy L, et al. Critical care nurse work environments 2018: findings and implications. Crit Care Nurse 2019;39(2):67–84.

32. Wong, K. 12 best practices for peer-to-peer recognition. August 12, 2023 at https://www.achievers.com/blog/peer-to-peer-recognition/. Accessed September 25, 2023.

33. DAISY Foundation at https://www.daisyfoundation.org/about-daisy-award. Ac-cessed September 25, 2023.

34. American Association of Critical Care Nurses. Beacon Award at https://www. aacn.org/nursing-excellence/beacon-awards?tab=Who%20Can%20Apply%3F. Accessed September 25, 2023.

35. Emergency Nurses Association. Lantern Award at https://www.ena.org/about/ awards-recognition/lantern. Accessed September 25, 2023.

36. Academy of Medical-Surgical Nurses. PRISM Award at https://amsn.org/Learning-Development/Awards/Unit-Award-AMSN-PRISM-Award. Accessed September 25, 2023.

37. Watkins, A., Valuing vs recognizing employees. April 22, 2015. Retrieved September 30, 2023 from: https://www.mediapartners.com/blog/post/valuing_vs_recognizing_ employees.

38. Kaufman T, Christensen J, Newton A. Employee performance: what causes great work? 2015. O.C.Tanner. www.octanner.com/content/dam/oc-tanner/documents/ whitepapers/2015_Cicero_WhitePaper_Drivers_of_Great_Work.pdf.

39. Harrison K. Why employee recognition is so important–and what you can do about it. Cutting Edge.2020 at https://cuttingedgepr.com/employeerecognition-important . Accessed September 25, 2023.

40. American Nurses Credentialing Center. Facts About Magnet Recognition Pro-gram at https://www.nursingworld.org/globalassets/organizational-programs/ magnet/magnet-factsheet.pdf. Accessed November 11, 2023.

41. Graystone R. The value of magnet recognition. J Nurs Adm 2019;49(10S Suppl):S1–3.

42. Dempsey C, Reilly BA. Nurse engagement: what are the contributing factors for success? 2016;21(1).

43. Dempsey C, Assi MJ. The impact of nurse engagement on quality, safety, and the experience of care: what nurse leaders should know. Nurs Adm Q 2018;42(3): 278–83. https://doi.org/10.1097/NAQ.0000000000000305.

44. Sherman R, Cohn T. When staff disengage. Am Nurse 2022;17:7 20–23.
45. O'Grady TP, Clavelle JT. Transforming shared governance: toward professional governance for nursing 2021;51(4):206–11.
46. Brennan D, Wendt L. Increasing quality and patient outcomes with staff engagement and shared governance. Online J Issues Nurs 2021;26(2).
47. Kutney-Lee A, Germack H, Hatfield L, et al. Nurse engagement in shared governance and patient and nurse outcomes. J Nurs Adm 2016;46(11):605–12.
48. Porter-O'Grady T. Principles for sustaining shared/professional governance in nursing. Nurs Manag 2019;0(1):36–41.
49. French-Bravo M, Crow G. Shared governance: the role of buy-in in bringing about change. Online J Issues Nurs 2015;20(2):8.

A Post-Pandemic Review of American Association of Critical Care Nurses's Domains of Establishing and Sustaining Healthy Work Environments

Strategies for Nurse Leaders

Ashley Waddell, PhD, RN, FAAN[a],*,
Amanda Stefancyk Oberlies, PhD, MBA, RN, FAAN[b]

KEYWORDS

- Nursing • Nurse leader • Healthy work environments • Wellbeing
- AACN's standards for establishing and sustaining healthy work environments

KEY POINTS

- American Association of Critical Care Nurses's Standards for Establishing and Sustaining Healthy Work Environments remain useful for nurse leaders to assess and plan interventions to improve work environments.
- Prioritizing wellbeing for members of the care team, and leaders, is essential for providing quality care.
- Nurse leaders can apply practical strategies to improve each domain within the Healthy Work Environment Standards.

INTRODUCTION

The coronavirus disease 2019 (COVID-19) pandemic has had a profound impact on health care providers, and the care delivery system. A significant nursing shortage, high-demand for nursing care, and financial challenges continue to complicate efforts to empower high-functioning teams that create high-quality patient outcomes. Efforts to re-build and strengthen healthy work environments are a priority in many organizations, but knowing where to start can feel overwhelming. This article explores current evidence and practical strategies for nurse leaders to advance a healthy work environment, using American Association of Critical Care Nurses's enduring Standards for

[a] Director Government Affairs and Educational Programs, Organization of Nurse Leaders MA, RI, CT, NH, VT; [b] Organization of Nurse Leaders MA, RI, CT, NH, VT
* Corresponding author. PO Box 178, Whitinsville, MA 01588.
E-mail address: awaddell@oonl.org

Crit Care Nurs Clin N Am 36 (2024) 367–377
https://doi.org/10.1016/j.cnc.2024.01.003
0899-5885/24/© 2024 Elsevier Inc. All rights reserved.
ccnursing.theclinics.com

Establishing and Sustaining Healthy Work Environments.[1] Authors propose adding the domain of Wellbeing to guide leaders in holistically addressing the health of all care team members and the work environment.

BACKGROUND

There is an unquestionable connection between nurse leaders, quality patient outcomes, staff retention, staff engagement, and healthy work environments.[2] Nurse leaders bring a variety of styles, strengths, skills, and approaches to their work, and how those come together has a lot to do with how well nursing teams function. First published nearly in 2005 and revised in 2016, the Standards for Establishing and Sustaining Healthy Work Environments[1] provides a framework that should (still) be top of mind for nurse leaders who are working tirelessly to re-build healthy work environments and address the multiple leadership demands including staffing, quality, safety, satisfaction, nurse retention, and engagement, just to name a few.[3]

Describing the early 2020s as a time of disruption for the United States nursing workforce would be a significant understatement. Multiple factors including an uptick in nurse retirements, resignations, requests to reduce hours, and competitive labor markets are leaving nurse leaders and organizations grappling with strategies to attract and retain staff, keep beds open, and guard against staff burnout.[4]

To understand the impact of the COVID-19 pandemic, The American Nurses Foundation conducted several Pulse Surveys with US nurses.[5] The most recently published data, reflecting responses from more than 11,000 nurses, paint a distressing picture: only 42% of the nurses feel that their work environments are healthy and positive. Nurses describe increasing instances of bullying and incivility coming from patients and families. Fifty-five percent of the responding nurses describe their units as being staffed with the appropriate number of nurses less than half of the time; 59% of the nurses report that they are asked daily or weekly to work more than their scheduled hours to cover unfilled shifts, and 49% of the direct care nurses either intend to leave their positions or consider leaving. Within the same survey, 31% of the nurses selected *"Genuinely listen to my voice and respond to my needs"* as one of the top approaches for nurse leaders to use to improve satisfaction.[5] Nursing leadership expert, Dr Rose Sherman, interprets the findings this way: "… our nurses are telling us what is happening today in their work environments is not sustainable moving forward. We must listen to them closely (without judgment) and ask for their ideas."[6] Similarly, Roso and colleagues identified a healthy work environment as a key to stabilizing the nursing workforce.[7]

Viewing nursing workforce changes through a different lens, Epic researchers, who analyze electronic health record data, studied 26 million shifts across 189 US health care organizations in 2021 and 2022 and reported a decrease in median nurse tenure by 19.5%, and the number of 12-hour shifts staffed by nurses new to the organization rose by 55.5%.[8] These data highlight an important new trend—clinical staff have far less experience today. Less tenure and more new nurses mean nurse leaders need to assess and respond to institutional and experiential knowledge that has been lost. The growing gaps in knowledge associated with these data should cause pause for nurse leaders, as a rise in safety and quality issues would not be surprising. How to address the growing gaps in knowledge associated with these data will require a thoughtful approach to recruitment, retention, culture, teamwork, policy, and practice.

NURSING LEADERSHIP AND HEALTHY WORK ENVIRONMENTS

Nursing leadership is the key to establishing and maintaining a healthy work environment. Seminal work on defining a healthy work environment is credited to the American

Association of Critical Care Nurses (AACN) and includes 6 evidence-based standards: effective decision-making, ture collaboration, appropriate staffing, authentic leadership, skilled communication, and meaningful recognition.[1] Since the first publication of AACN's Standards for Establishing and Sustaining Healthy Work Environments in 2005, the six standards have been extensively studied and remain unchanged. Within this evidence-based framework, each standard is considered essential, see **Box 1**.[1]

This framework focuses on interpersonal relationships and professional performance. Collectively, the six standards—plus wellbeing, should inform how nurse leaders approach quality, safety, health, and satisfaction in their units and with their teams. We will discuss current evidence and practical strategies that can help nurse leaders build and sustain healthy work environments.

EFFECTIVE DECISION-MAKING

This domain of AACN's Establishing and Sustaining Healthy Work Environments framework describes the critical role nurses must play in policy, directing and evaluating care delivery, and leading clinical and organizational operations (p.5).[1] Nurse leaders are critical in all aspects of this standard, but even the most skilled leaders have been challenged by conditions during and in the aftermath of the pandemic. Established practices and norms that existed before the pandemic, such as participation in nursing councils and shared decision-making, need to be revitalized in many organizations.[9] Conditions such as inadequate staffing, high turnover, and persistent on-boarding have made it difficult for nurses to contribute beyond direct care provision. Similarly, leaders are balancing competing demands of staffing, ensuring conditions for safe and effective practice, budget challenges, and limited time they can spend on supporting domains of professional practice.

Nurse leaders must work diligently to make it possible for clinical nurses to be empowered in their practice. Clinical nurses must feel supported in delivering care to patients and communities and must have a voice in policy and practice decisions.

Box 1
The standards for establishing and sustaining healthy work environments—plus wellbeing

Effective Decision-Making: Nurses must be valued and committed partners in making policy, directing and evaluating clinical care, and leading organizational operations.

True Collaboration: Nurses must be relentless in pursuing and fostering true collaboration.

Appropriate Staffing: Staffing must ensure the effective match between patient needs and nurse competencies.

Authentic Leadership: Nurse leaders must fully embrace the imperative of a healthy work environment, authentically live it, and engage others in its achievement.

Skilled Communication: Nurses must be as proficient in communication skills as they are in clinical skills.

Meaningful Recognition: Nurses must be recognized and must recognize others for the value each brings to the work of the organization.

[a] *Wellbeing*: Wellbeing must be a priority. Focus is required to support individual wellbeing as well as creating an environment that promotes wellness, team function, and quality patient outcomes.

[a]Not part of the AACN framework.

American Association of Critical-Care Nurses. ([AACN], 2016).

Participation in decision-making can be accomplished through professional governance models. "Nursing Professional Governance is defined as the profession of nursing's control and ownership over decisions and actions related to nursing practice, quality, competence, and knowledge management."[(p217)9] When thinking about how to revitalize professional governance models following the pandemic, leaders may want to consider the 3 fundamental principles of Professional Governance offered by Porter-O'Grady and Pappas: (1) it must be grounded in accountability at the practice level, (2) structures must enable and support clinical decision-making, and (3) the same structures must enable distributive decision-making (2022).[9] Nurse leaders must develop skills that are grounded in equity, with a commitment to elevating the perspectives of direct care providers.[10] Different structures can effect decision-making on units, within departments, and organizations. Leaders should consider the extent to which members of their team have an opportunity to contribute to decisions. Leaders must also work to cultivate a culture of ethical practice—including giving voice to all stakeholders, reducing hierarchies to improve collaboration, and addressing victimization to move toward principled moral agency.[(pS29)11]

TRUE COLLABORATION

The domain of *true collaboration* is best expressed as a deep passion and commitment to fostering relationships, teamwork, and collaboration.[(p. 4)1] To some extent the pandemic stimulated improved collaboration. Whether sharing clinical best practices or sharing resources, clinicians, teams, and organizations worked together in new and collaborative ways during the COVID-19 pandemic. Professional organizations also served in the important role as convener, creating space for members to share ideas and resources and offer support to one another.[12] "Trust is what helps navigate boundaries and creates a sense that everyone is doing his/her part to serve patients, with each working within his/her professional scope of responsibility."[(p. 220)9] Collaboration, trust, and teamwork come together to create an environment where nurses can feel valued for their contributions and supported when they encounter challenges.

In practice, true collaboration can take different forms. Some nurse leaders are explicit in trying to hire team players, asking job applicants to describe experiences of working on a team and ask them for specific examples of how they backed up other team members in prior jobs or while in school.[13] "Building strong team backup is critical to staff retention. Team inclusion is a vital aspect of building psychological safety."[13] Some leaders make it clear that teamwork is a job expectation, while others integrate it into daily practice on their units. Implementing a battle-buddies program is an example of a moving a strategy from military training into health care. The idea is simple—nurses can sign-up for, or are assigned, a partner to help each other get through the day.[14] Intentionally designing structures that hard-wire teamwork and collaboration have always been important, but now, in times of workforce instability, they are essential.

APPROPRIATE STAFFING

The domain of *appropriate staffing* addresses the importance of matching patient needs with nurse competencies. "When patients' characteristics and nurses' competencies match and synergize, outcomes for the patient are optimal." (p. 64)[15]

Nurse leaders work tirelessly to ensure the right mix of staff is available to provide care. Many dimensions are considered when making decisions about how to optimally assign nurses to patients during a shift. These dimensions are articulated in The Synergy Model and include 3 components: "patients' characteristics of concern to nurses,

nurses' competencies important to patients, and patients' outcomes that result when patients' characteristics and nurses' competencies are mutually enhancing." (p. 64)[15] This model is operationalized through a thoughtful and deliberate process in which nurse leaders assign nurses to patients. Nurse leaders consider the skills and competencies of the nurse, years of experience, as well as additional duties such as teaching or orienting. They consider patient characteristics such as expected interventions and workload anticipated during the future shift, social and family involvement, spiritual needs, and interdisciplinary involvement. Additional considerations include other members of the care team, proximity of patients on a unit, plans for discharge or transfer.

Many issues make achieving appropriate staffing a challenge, especially following the COVID-19 pandemic. The intersection of a highly competitive labor market, nursing shortage, nurse burnout, increased demand for health care services, and financial stress within the health care system all impact the delivery of nursing services. Additionally, nurses are rightly seeking competitive compensation, better work environments, safe nurse staffing, and moral leadership.[16] When advocating for appropriate staffing resources, nurse leaders should focus on clearly articulating patient needs, quality outcomes, and team member wellbeing. The work environment must be viewed in totality and addressed in a holistic manner because inadequate staffing contributes to stress, exhaustion, and burnout for both nurses and nurse leaders, and interventions to improve wellbeing, and—by extension—patient outcomes, must address both staff and leadership.[17,18] Workload is a big driver of dissatisfaction and nurses should be able to come to work without feelings of dread and leave their shift feeling satisfied.

Advancing Professional Governance, cultivating collaboration, and supporting wellbeing and professional practice will require intentionality. Necessary nurse leader attributes will be explored next.

AUTHENTIC LEADERSHIP

The domain of *authentic leadership* centers around a genuine commitment to work toward, and engage others in, building healthy work environments. "Authentic leaders act upon their values and beliefs while transparently interacting with others."[2] The presence of authentic nurse leadership was positively associated with health work environments in 2 studies performed during the COVID-19 pandemic.[7,19] Authentic leadership has been shown to have a negative correlation to turnover intention, suggesting that "when nursing leaders sincerely care for nurses, listen to their opinions, respect members, and provide care, turnover intentions can be reduced." (p. 2182)[20]

For leaders interested in better understanding authentic leadership, The Authentic Nurse Leadership framework has 3 main constructs—personal integrity, transparency, and altruism, with 5 supporting attributes: moral ethical courage, self-awareness, relationship integrality, shared decision-making, and caring.[2] This framework can be used to reflect upon personal areas of strength and potential for future growth. Authentic leaders bring "awareness, truth, and presence to interactions.[21]

Listening is a nurse leader superpower. Sherman[21] suggests working on listening and self-reflection, seeking feedback from peers, and building relationships, including with mentors, to grow as an authentic leader. Some leaders find it helpful to seek feedback from colleagues about their professional presence. Pappas describes nurse leaders as "compassionate professionals, accountable to how we behave and interact, make decisions, and lead." (p. 362)[22] She calls on nurse leaders to make the workplace a contributor to clinician wellbeing by focusing on the relational, or humanistic aspects of work, and facilitating structures to create a sense of community.[23]

SKILLED COMMUNICATION

The domain of *skilled communication* reflects the critical importance of having good communication skills. Communication skills are linked with quality and safety, team performance, and patient satisfaction. Younger generations in the workplace are more comfortable with text communication, and in-person dialogue can feel uncomfortable. In response, organizations recognize that they need to do more to build communication skills among members of their teams so that important information is accurately shared and acted upon, and so colleagues can address conflict and support one another. Many organizations are now teaching communication skills as part of orientation and yearly competency reviews (Sherman, 2023).[23]

In practice, nurses regularly update patients and families and can share information that will help them make decisions.[24] Nurse leaders can model clear, concise, and respectful communication, and they should coach members of their team to do the same. Establishing ground rules and expectations for communication during huddles and handoffs can also help to empower staff, reduce perceived hierarchies, and guide communication.[25] Effective communication requires both sharing and receiving information. Developing listening skills is equally important when working to improve communication. Nurse leaders can conduct listening tours and hold forums to openly discuss important topics. Stay interviews are another format for dialogue in which nurse leaders can learn what is working well and what can be improved, from the perspective of new and tenured employees.[26] Lastly, it is important for nurse leaders to seek continuing leadership development and to support the professional development of members of their team. Engaging with professional nursing organizations is another key consideration for both nurse leaders and clinical nurses. Many professional nursing organizations offer educational programming designed to fit the needs of their members as well as providing opportunities to connect with a network of colleagues.

MEANINGFUL RECOGNITION

The domain of *meaningful recognition* focuses on the importance of recognizing nurses and others for the significant and unique contributions they make to the organization. It serves as a mechanism for sharing positive feedback and driving engagement. The recognition should be personal, strengths-based, and specific, and it should acknowledge how one person's actions impact the work of the team and the outcomes of the patient. The recognition should also be provided in a timely manner. "When done right, recognition boosts engagement and strengthens connections between people and across the company."[(p. 2)27]

Gallup conducted a large-scale study across multiple industries, hundreds of organizations, and thousands of teams to explore the relationship between recognition and employee outcomes. The study findings reveal multiple reasons leaders and organizations should recognize contributions of team members. Among the most important for nursing leaders, the study results suggest employee recognition has a substantial impact on safety incidents. Study authors explain the relationship this way: recognition builds social bonds, and "When social bonds are strong, people look out for one another. They do things the right way, not because the rules say so, but because they don't want to see the people they care about get hurt."[(p. 7)27] Recognition communicates "you matter", and it affirms the value of doing quality work. It is important for nurse leaders to be concrete and action-oriented when it comes to meaningful recognition.

Three focus areas of meaningful recognition are identified by Sweeney & Wiseman and include (1) reasonable payment for level of service provided; (2) public recognition within the organization and the profession; and (3) opportunities for professional development."[(p81)28] Each of these focus areas can guide unit and organizational strategies for meaningful recognition.

Whether sparked by the COVID-19 pandemic or not, nurses are aware of their value and have become more transactional, advocating for higher wages, increased flexibility, and bonus pay.[29] Leaders should use conversations about wages to discuss total compensation, inclusive of health and retirement benefits, tuition reimbursement, and other offerings included in the benefit package. Organizations have likely conducted several recent market analyses to determine how their salaries and benefits compare with competitors. As a complement, listening tours may provide useful insight if an organization wants to better understand what meaningful benefits look like through an employee perspective. Additionally, it may be useful to account for the cost of housing and childcare, availability of transportation, safety in the vicinity of the organization, and the burden of debt among employees to better understand social and financial pain-points from the perspective of staff. Armed with information, organizations should work to more clearly articulate the value of the employee benefit packages and consider offering financial planning and loan forgiveness guidance to employees. Some organizations have flexed their benefit options to address what's valued by different generations in the workforce. For example, younger employees who are staying on their parents' health care benefits may not need or value health care benefits but would really benefit from loan forgiveness options or increased tuition reimbursement. At the unit level, charge nurse pay, preceptor pay, overtime pay, and so on, should be considered in the context of appreciating members of the team who step up, and do more.

Public recognition can be accomplished in many ways. One great example is the DAISY Award, designed to celebrate nurses who are nominated by patients, families, and colleagues. The DAISY Award is an evidence-based program that has been associated with improved job satisfaction, retention rate, teamwork, pride, organizational culture, and a positive work environment.[30] The DAISY Foundation partners with thousands of organizations to offer recognition to nurses.

Professional nursing organizations also offer many awards to recognize excellence in practice, education, research, innovation, and leadership, just to name a few. The nominations can take time to pull together and write, so many nurse leaders find it helpful to make notes throughout the year if they plan to nominate a colleague for a professional award. Nurses Week celebrations within organizations frequently include awards to recognize excellence among the nursing team. Once you start looking, you will likely find many ways to recognize members of the team for their great work, now make nominating them a priority!

Providing opportunities and budgeting for indirect time to support professional development for members of your team communicates 2 important messages. It reiterates "you matter" and "you are doing good work", and "we as an organization want to support you in advancing your knowledge and skills". When nurse leaders make professional development opportunities available to their team, it demonstrates a commitment to the growth and advancement of individuals, as well as the collective team.

Nurse leaders should discuss professional goals with staff during their annual review, and more often, as indicated. Newer nurses may need a supportive nudge or mentorship to attend a professional meeting, as this might be a new experience. Funds should be allocated at the unit, program, or department level to support professional development. Savvy nurse leaders will have a sense of what types of programs they would like to see members of their team attend, and they should use the need for new skills or competencies in the team as an opportunity to develop their staff.

Planning is important—thinking ahead to what the next year will look will help leaders plan professional development to help the team succeed. For organizations that offer tuition reimbursement, staff may need help navigating the policies to access the funding, and leaders should support staff in accessing this benefit. Last, but not least, advancing education, certification, and job promotions should all be celebrated.

WELLBEING—A DOMAIN NOT EXPLICITLY IN AMERICAN ASSOCIATION OF CRITICAL CARE NURSES'S STANDARDS FOR ESTABLISHING AND SUSTAINING HEALTHY WORK ENVIRONMENTS

While not explicitly covered in the AACN framework for healthy work environments, employee wellbeing cannot be overlooked. In 2017, the National Academy of Medicine (NAM) launched an Action Collaborative on Clinician Wellbeing and Resilience. "Clinician wellbeing supports improved patient-clinician relationships, a high-functioning care team, and an engaged and effective workforce." (n.p)[31] Their website provides links to resources and evidence-based best practices, these and other resources can be found at https://nam.edu/clinicianwellbeing/. The Wellbeing at Work Framework[32] is a comprehensive and evidence-based framework that is useful for leaders to apply for a holistic approach to team-member wellbeing. This framework includes 5 tenets of wellbeing (Career, Social, Financial, Physical, and Community). Nurse leaders can use these tenets to holistically explore wellbeing with members of their team and make strides to improve wellbeing at work.

Addressing wellness at work is also a contributor in employment decisions. Generation Z and Millennial nurses are identifying organizational commitment to wellbeing as a priority when seeking employment.[14] Organizations should have a process to assess and address physical, emotional, and psychological wellbeing.[10] According to Melnyk,[18] nurses had better mental and physical health outcomes when they perceived that their workplace supported their health. If bullying and incivility is present, it must be addressed. At alarming rates, nurses are reporting bullying and incivility from patients and families,[5] and it is impacting their mental health and wellbeing. Some organizations are increasing signage and communication with patients and families about appropriate behaviors. In Massachusetts, hospitals adopted a united code of conduct to protect workers from escalating violence and harassment.[33]

Nurse leaders must focus on individual wellbeing as well as creating an environment that supports wellness, team function, and quality patient outcomes. Care team members all have a role in reducing mental health stigma so that clinicians feel safe in seeking help if they are suffering from burnout, depression, or suicidal ideation.[18] Nurse leaders should be intentional about what changes they can make in the unit to enhance the multiple tenets of wellbeing, and engaging team members in the effort would be even better. Attention is needed to refine workflows to allow nurses more time with patients and more opportunities to engage in professional actions that cultivate professional joy and satisfaction. Nurse leaders should consider the evidence and look into eliminating 12-hour shifts as they are associated with negative impact on nurses' physical and mental health as well as a contributor to unsafe care.[17] Nursing teams should work together and prioritize getting everyone a shift break. The wellbeing of nurses, team members and leaders must be prioritized when building or enhancing a healthy work environment.

SUMMARY

Nurse leaders can influence culture, communication practices, staffing decisions, and outcomes by addressing the domains of a healthy work environment. AACN's

Standards for Establishing and Sustaining Healthy Work Environments can be used to help focus efforts to reconnect clinical teams with meaningful and satisfying work. Collectively, the 6 standards—plus wellbeing—should inform how nurse leaders approach quality, safety, health, and satisfaction in their units and with their teams. The past several years have demonstrated that there are many aspects of health care delivery that are beyond the control of any individual, and challenges from the pandemic will persist, including the nursing shortage, reimbursement shortfalls, and increasing demand for nursing and health care services. Nurse leaders can control how they "show up," how they lead, and how they advocate for their teams. They are encouraged to use the evidence and pragmatic leadership strategies presented in this article to reflect on the current health of their team, their work environment, and to consider targeted areas for investment and improvement.

CLINICS CARE POINTS

- Healthy work environments are built and maintained with focused strategies. Best practice stratgies are shared.
- The AACN Standards for Establishing and Substaining Health Work Environments should guide leaders and staff in efforts to improve work environments.
- The wellbeing of all team members, including leadres, should be prioritized.

DISCLOSURE

Both authors have no conflicts of interest to disclose.

REFERENCES

1. American Association of Critical-Care Nurses [AACN]. AACN standards for establishing and sustaining healthy work environments: a journey to excellence. 2nd edition. Aliso Viejo, CA,: American Association of Critical-Care Nurses; 2016. Available at: https://www.aacn.org/wd/hwe/docs/hwestandards.pdf.
2. Giordano-Mulligan M, Eckardt S. Authentic nurse leadership Conceptual framework: nurses' Perception of authentic nurse leader attributes. Nurs Adm Q 2019;43(2):164–74.
3. Dimino K, Learmonth AE, Fajardo CC. Nurse Managers leading the way: Reenvisioning stress to Maintain healthy work environments. Crit Care Nurse 2021;41(5):52–8.
4. Organization of Nurse Leaders. The Nursing Workforce Challenges and Solutions During the COVID Era. 4. The Organization of Nurse Leaders. Published January 2022. Available at: https://onl.memberclicks.net/assets/docs/ONLWorkforce ReportJan2022/ONL_Nursing_Workforce_Report_Jan_2022.pdf.
5. American Nurses Foundation. Pulse on the Nation's nurses survey series: 2022 workplace survey nurses not feeling heard, ongoing staffing and workplace issues contributing to unhealthy work environment. Silver Spring, MD: American Nurses Foundation; 2022. Available at: https://www.nursingworld.org/~4a209f/globalassets/covid19/anf-2022-workforce-written-report-final.pdf.
6. Sherman R. The Current Pulse of the Nursing Workforce. Blog post. Published August 11, 2022. Available at: https://emergingrnleader.com/the-current-pulse-on-rn-emotions-about-work/. Accessed December 15, 2023.

7. Roso R, Fitzpatrick J, Masick K. Perceptions of US nurses and nurse leaders on authentic nurse leadership, healthy work environment, intent to leave and nurse well-being during a second pandemic year: a cross sectional study. J Nurs Manag 2022;30(7):2699–706.

8. Thayer J, Zillmer J, Sandberg N, Miller AR, Nagel P, MacGibbon A. 'The New Nurse' Is the New Normal. Epic Research. Available at: https://epicresearch.org/articles/the-new-nurse-is-the-new-normal. Published on June 2, 2022. Accessed on December 15, 2023. https://epicresearch.org/articles/the-new-nurse-is-the-new-normal.

9. Porter-O'Grady T, Pappas S. Professional governance in a time of crisis. J Nurs Adm 2022;52(4):217–21.

10. Porter-O'Grady T. Abandoning Blue-Collar management: leading nursing professionals into a new Age for practice. Nurs Adm Q 2023;47(3):200–8.

11. Rushton C. Creating a culture of ethical practice in health care delivery systems. Hastings Center Report. Special Report: Nurses at the Table: Nursing, Ethics, and Healthy Policy. September-October 2016: S28-31.

12. Organization of Nurse Leaders MA, RI, CT, NH, VT. The nursing workforce report: Challenges and solutions during the COVID era. January 2022. Available at: https://onl.memberclicks.net/assets/docs/ONLWorkforceReportJan2022/ONL_Nursing_Workforce_Report_Jan_2022.pdf. Accessed December 4, 2023.

13. Sherman R. Rebuilding a Culture of Team Backup. Blog post. Published August 22, 2022. Available at: https://emergingrnleader.com/rebuilding-a-culture-of-team-backup/. Accessed December 5, 2023.

14. Sherman R. The business case for nurse wellbeing. Blog post. Published on May 13, 2021. Available at: https://emergingrnleader.com/the-business-case-for-nurse-wellbeing/. Accessed December 5, 2023.

15. Curley M. Patient-nurse synergy: Optimizing patient outcomes. Am J Crit Care 1998;7(1):64–72.

16. Boston-Leary K, Stone B. The nursing profession circa 2030. Nursing 2022; 52(12):34–9.

17. Melnyk BM. Making an evidence-based case for urgent action to address clinician burnout. American Journal of Accountable Care 2019;7(2):12–4.

18. Melnyk BM. Burnout, depression and Suicide in nurses/clinicians and Learners: an urgent call for action to enhance professional well-being and healthcare safety. Worldviews Evid Based Nurs 2020;17(1):2–5.

19. Raso R, Fitzpatrick JJ, Masick K, et al. Perceptions of authentic nurse leadership and work environment and the pandemic impact for nurse leaders and clinical nurses. J Nurs Adm 2021;51(5):257–63.

20. Hwang J, Song EK, Ko S. Relationships among basic psychological needs, organizational commitment, perceived authentic leadership and turnover intention in Korean nurses: a cross-sectional study. J Nurs Manag 2022;30(7):2176–84.

21. Sherman R. Become an authentic leader. Blog post. Published on April 1, 2019. Available at: https://emergingrnleader.com/becoming-an-authentic-leader/. Accessed December 4, 2023.

22. Pappas S. The role of nurse leaders in the well-being of clinicians. J Nurs Adm 2021;51(7/8):362–3.

23. This is 24: Sherman, R. Helping nurses with communication skills. Blog post. Published on July 13, 2023. Available at: https://emergingrnleader.com/helping-nurses-with-communication-skills/. Accessed December 4, 2023.

24. Dees ML, Carpenter JS, Longtin K. Communication between Registered nurses and family members of Intensive care Unit patients. Crit Care Nurse 2022; 42(6):25–34.

25. Njambi M, Rawson H, Redley B. A brief intervention to standardize postanesthetic clinical handoff. Nurs Health Sci 2021;23(1):219–26.
26. Sherman, R. Do stay interviews now with your new graduates. Blog post. Published on September 7, 2023. Available at: https://emergingrnleader.com/do-stay-interviews-now-with-your-new-graduate-nurses/. Accessed December 4, 2023.
27. Gallup (2023). From praise to profits: The business case for recognition at work. Available at: https://dcu001bswmooj.cloudfront.net/s3fs-public/2023-09/from-praise-to-profits-the-business-case-for-recognition-at-work.pdf%20gallup.pdf. Accessed December 4, 2023.
28. Sweeney CD, Wiseman R. Retaining the best recognizing what meaningful recognition is to Nurses as a Strategy for Nurse Leaders. J Nurs Adm 2023;53(2):81–7.
29. Sherman R. Helping nurses with financial wellbeing. Blog post. Published on December 1, 2022. Available at: https://emergingrnleader.com/helping-nurses-with-financial-wellbeing/. Accessed December 10, 2023.
30. The DAISY Foundation. About the DAISY Award. 2023. Available at: https://www.daisyfoundation.org/about-daisy-award. Accessed December 10, 2023.
31. National Academy of Medicine. (2022). Action collaborative on clinician well-being and resilience. Available at: https://nam.edu/initiatives/clinician-resilience-and-well-being/. Accessed December 4, 2023.
32. Clifton J, Harter J. Wellbeing at work. Washington, DC: Gallup Press; 2021.
33. Kayser A. Massachusetts hospitals adopt united code of conduct to combat workplace violence. Becker's Hospital Review. Published January 30, 2023. Available at: https://www.beckershospitalreview.com/workforce/massachusetts-hospitals-adopt-united-code-of-conduct-to-combat-workplace-violence.html. Accessed December 4, 2023.

Support for Clinical Nurse Educators
Imparting Key Leadership Skills

Jennifer Barsamian, DNP, RN, NPD-C[a], Kerry Carnevale, DNP, RN[b],*

KEYWORDS

- Clinical nurse educator • CNE • Unit based educator • Bedside clinical educator
- UBE • Unit-based educator professional development

KEY POINTS

- Supporting the transition of clinical nurses to a clinical nurse educator (CNE) leadership role is not well described in the literature.
- Transition to a CNE role without orientation, including essential communication skills, contributes to role ambiguity and increased stress.
- Education focused on essential communication skills increases CNE comfort with initiating difficult conversations.

INTRODUCTION

Clinical nurse educator (CNE) responsibilities include orientation, competency assessment and management, clinical practice support, role modeling, and mentoring of nurses involved in direct patient care.[1] The CNE role varies across organizations in terms of title, role description, and educational preparation. At the site of this Quality Improvement (QI) project, the role is titled Unit Based Educator and staff nurses are selected for their clinical acumen, however, they do not receive any standard and formal training to prepare them for this role transition. Many CNEs have cited public speaking, peer education, difficult conversations, constructive feedback, and conflict management as areas in which they struggle within their professional practice. These perceived and actual knowledge gaps can persist well into their practice as CNEs.

Assuming a formal leadership role on the unit can be a socially isolating experience that sets the CNE apart from their previous peer group of staff nurses. As their work is mainly unit based, their daily interaction with their CNE peer group is often restricted. This isolation and shift in role definition can compound the difficulties of role transition.

[a] Mount Auburn Hospital, 330 Mount Auburn Street, Cambridge, MA 02138, USA; [b] Beth Israel Deaconess Medical Center, 330 Brookline Avenue, Boston, MA 02215, USA
* Corresponding author.
E-mail address: kcarneva@bidmc.harvard.edu

Crit Care Nurs Clin N Am 36 (2024) 379–391
https://doi.org/10.1016/j.cnc.2024.03.001
0899-5885/24/© 2024 Elsevier Inc. All rights reserved.
ccnursing.theclinics.com

Formal opportunities to collaborate, support, and learn from other CNEs in their role are, at times, limited. Clinical nurse educators participate in the planning and execution of educational and professional development opportunities for other nurses, but there are very few opportunities provided within our medical center that address their particular professional development needs. These knowledge deficits, a lack of focused development opportunities, and the experience of social isolation have a negative impact on CNEs' job satisfaction.

LITERATURE REVIEW

There is a paucity of literature documenting the transition from bedside nursing to a hospital-based role centered on the education of registered nurses practicing at the bedside.[2] Barriers and facilitators of transitioning from clinical practice to academia or from the role of the registered nurse to that of an advanced practice nurse are better documented[2,3,4]; however, it is important to note that those role changes involve formal education and training in the form of advanced degrees and/or certifications. The role transition from expert registered nurse to novice CNE at our organization is not preceded by formal and focused preparation or required academic and/or professional certification.

In addition to ensuring nursing staff clinical competence, essential CNE skills include leading practice and policy change, identifying opportunities for QI, and providing colleagues performance feedback using strong communication skills.[2,3] In a small qualitative study examining the challenges associated with transitioning from the role of staff nurse to clinical educator, Manning and Neville[5] identified minimal orientation to the role, lack of role clarity, and being underprepared for the responsibilities to the clinical educator role as contributing to increased stress in clinical educators. The absence of a standardized orientation to the clinical educator role contributes to new educators feeling overwhelmed or unconfident with role related skills including education planning and delivery, and experiencing role ambiguity.[6]

Successful transition from expert clinician to bedside clinical educator requires dedicated orientation and mentorship to support socialization to the new role and clinical educator skills acquisition.[5] Clear, well-defined clinical educator role expectations, coupled with mentoring, focused on role transition, and development of essential educator skills assist clinical educators with the transition to their new role.[6] Additionally, a formal CNE orientation, continuing education opportunities, and establishing peer group connections can improve role satisfaction by reducing role isolation and improving role clarity.[7] Collaborative clinical educator practice provides opportunities for shared resources, professional development, and role socialization, which may improve role satisfaction and job retention.[7]

The aforementioned gap in the literature regarding the role of the CNE, combined with documented transitional challenges for nurses making other role transitions without the benefit of formal training and preparation, highlight the need for this QI project. The purpose of this article is to describe and analyze the effectiveness of an educational intervention to improve CNE comfort with conducting difficult conversations, providing constructive feedbacks, and conducting an effective debrief.

DESIGN/METHODS

Approximately 40 CNEs, representing all unit types from inpatient and ambulatory practice areas, were invited via email to complete a communication skills needs assessment survey. Based on these results, a targeted educational intervention entitled *Courageous Communication* was developed as the authors' Doctor of Nursing

Practice QI project. This series included 3 in person, peer protected sessions for focused learning, and social connection for CNEs, as well as a secure and online virtual community. The online community was limited to the facilitators and CNE participants and was designed to provide additional resources and opportunities for support, discussion, and continued interaction as participants put theory into practice between sessions.

The CNEs received a second email describing the content for each session and an invitation to register for the sessions. As the content was unique to each session, CNEs were not required to attend all 3 sessions in order to participate in the educational intervention. To ensure participant confidentiality the initial needs assessment surveys, post session evaluations, and final series evaluation were collected and managed in REDCap data capture tools, a secure and reliable online database.[8]

Setting

This QI project was completed at a large and urban academic medical center. In the organization, more than 40 CNEs practice across the medical center in a wide range of specialty units.

Needs Assessment

Clinical nurse educators have anecdotally articulated a struggle with role transition, particularly in relation to non-clinical skills, including teaching strategies, giving feedback, and having difficult conversations. It was important to take a critical look at the knowledge gap by allowing the members of the group to identify and prioritize their learning-related needs. The needs assessment tool for this QI project was developed utilizing issues identified in the literature and the authors' personal experiences. It was then reviewed by a Doctorate faculty advisor, the medical center's nNurse sScientist, and was shared with colleagues to ensure content clarity.

The needs assessment was designed to capture self-identified educational needs, learning priorities, connections to their CNE peer group, and unit leadership and comfort of CNEs, specifically related to navigating difficult conversations and providing feedbacks. A link to survey questions was emailed to CNEs via REDCap and included 24 5-point Likert scale items rating comfort level both with giving and receiving feedback, teaching small and large groups. As mentoring and peer support are essential elements of a successful transition to the CNE role,[2] questions were included to evaluate their level of connection to their CNE colleagues and unit leadership teams. Interestingly, free text responses in the initial needs assessment identified a knowledge gap related to conducting an effective debrief. As questions on this topic had not been included on the initial needs assessment, a supplemental needs assessment with 5 Likert scale items focused on comfort level in debriefing stressful incidents, simulation, and clinical scenarios was completed by participants prior to the final educational session.

Educational Sessions

The full educational series consisted of 3 2-hour sessions held more than an 8 week period. Content of these sessions was developed based on CNE responses to the initial needs assessment and were delivered by both authors via PowerPoint presentation, review of case studies, and group discussion. To accommodate the realities of life during the COVID-19 pandemic, each session was conducted by both authors multiple times in safe and socially distant small groups. Session 1 focused on difficult conversations and included didactic material on tips and strategies for initiating and navigating challenges with difficult conversations. Group discussions were centered on relevant case-based scenarios and participant raised examples. These scenarios provided a timely opportunity for CNEs to reflect on their experiences as leaders on the front line of the COVID-19 surge.

Session 2 was centered on giving and receiving feedback. The in person session included tips and strategies for providing, soliciting, and receiving constructive feedback, as well as relevant case-based scenarios. Participants also raised examples from their own practice and identified how feedback promotes teamwork and enhances safe patient care.

Session 3 was focused on conducting an effective debrief. The session provided education on techniques for initiating debriefs following stressful events on their unit and debriefing simulation and clinical scenarios to support staff education. Participants discussed their experiences with debriefs in their practice area. Institutional resources for staff resilience and trauma recovery were reviewed.

Online Community

To encourage clinical reflection, continued discussion and learning between sessions and provide more longitudinal support to participants, a secure and interactive online community was created on the institution's learning management system. Access to the online forum was restricted to participants and facilitators of the *Courageous Communication* series. Participants were encouraged to post about their experiences utilizing newly learned communication techniques between sessions and to solicit feedback and support with challenging situations from their peers. Facilitators provided links to relevant articles and additional resources related to each session topic on the community forum. Participation in the community was not mandatory.

Program Evaluation

Post session and series evaluation surveys were developed using a 5-point Likert scale as part of this QI project to evaluate participant learning and satisfaction. A link to an electronic survey-based evaluation was emailed via REDCap to participants following their completion of each learning session. The link to a final full program evaluation was emailed to participants who had attended at least 1 of the individual sessions, 1 week after the final live learning session to evaluate learner satisfaction with each element of the intervention including live sessions and the online community forum.

RESULTS
Quantitative Analysis

Descriptive statistics were used to characterize the QI participant demographics. Continuous variables were reported as means plus minus standard deviations. Categorical variables were reported as counts with frequencies. Fisher's exact test was performed to compare the differences in survey responses. P-values less than 0.05 were considered statistically significant.

Attendance for each of the 3 sessions ranged from 26 to 29 participants. Individual session post-survey response rates were sustained across the series. Twenty-seven CNEs attended Session 1 Difficult Conversations, and the post survey response rate was 81.5% (n = 22). Twenty-nine CNEs attended Session 2 Feedback, and the post survey response rate was 93% (n = 27). Twenty-six CNEs attended Session 3 Debriefs, and the post survey response rate was 84.6% (n = 22). There were a total of 30 unique participants in this series; the final series evaluation response rate was 73.3% (n = 22). The survey participants were similar in baseline characteristics. The majority of survey participants were on average aged 42 years to 45 years, had more than 15 years working as a nurse, had less than 4 years of experience as a CNE, practiced primarily in the medical surgical areas, and held a Bachelor's degree (**Table 1**).

The initial needs assessment survey guided the development of the content for the educational sessions. Clinical nurse educators identified the need for education related to initiating difficult conversations with peers about clinical practice issues, how to provide timely and meaningful feedback, and identifying situations when debriefing would be appropriate.

There were statistically significant differences between the needs assessment and Session 1 survey responses (**Table 2**). Participants were more comfortable initiating difficult conversations with their peers on the unit after participating in the session and managing conflict. No significant shift in answers was found on the feedback session questionnaire.

Participants had similar levels of comfort in providing constructive feedback to new nurses and to experienced staff nurses, and asking for feedback from peers. As the majority of participants already recognized the importance of debriefing after stressful events prior to educational intervention, there was no change in survey response. However, after Session 3, participants were more comfortable initiating debrief after a stressful event and were also more familiar with available resources to support staff with managing the effects of exposure to stressful events. Clinical nurse educators' answers consistently shifted toward "somewhat agree" and "strongly agree" in questions about the importance of debriefing non-critical events and feeling comfortable with debriefing non-critical events, but the differences were not statistically significant.

There was no statistically significant change between the initial needs assessment survey and the final series evaluation survey responses. Participants felt they had adequate opportunity to connect and strong collegial relationships with CNE colleagues. They felt valued as members of the nursing leadership on their unit and within the institution. Participants reported similar CNE workgroup attendance prior to and at the end of the educational series.

Qualitative Analysis

Content analysis was performed on responses to open-ended questions included in each live session post-survey evaluation and in the final survey at the summary of the sessions. The following four themes emerged from post-session evaluations and the summative program evaluation. Similar themes have been identified in prior studies including transition into a unit leadership role causing stress in interpersonal relationships with their former peer group, the value of connecting with an experienced CNE mentor into the role, the value of a formalized orientation to the role, and prioritization of their professional development.[2,5,7]

The value of peer interactions
Throughout the sessions, participants frequently expressed the importance of small group discussion with peers to support their professional development. Several participants expressed relief with the revelation that other CNEs were experiencing similar feelings of stress with approaching difficult conversations.

I was also relieved knowing that this is an issue all educators struggle with. As a novice educator, the advice from senior educators is extremely beneficial to my personal growth.

The sharing of experiences and problem solving to navigate challenges in role identity, to feel empowered to have a crucial conversation, and to network with their CNE peers and develop relationships for future professional support was recognized.

Table 1
Baseline participant characteristics

	Needs Assessment (n = 37)	Session 1 (n = 22)	Session 2 (n = 27)	Debrief Needs Assessment (n = 27)	Session 3 (n = 22)	Series Evaluation (n = 22)
Age, years	44 (11)	42 (10)	45 (10)	44 (10)	45 (11)	43 (9)
Years of experience as a nurse						
5–6	2 (5%)	0 (0%)	0 (0%)	0 (0%)	0 (0%)	0 (0%)
7–8	4 (11%)	3 (14%)	3 (11%)	3 (11%)	1 (5%)	3 (14%)
9–10	2 (5%)	3 (14%)	3 (11%)	3 (11%)	3 (14%)	2 (9%)
11–12	4 (11%)	0 (0%)	1 (4%)	2 (7%)	1 (5%)	0 (0%)
13–14	5 (14%)	5 (23%)	4 (15%)	5 (19%)	5 (23%)	5 (23%)
≥15	20 (54%)	11 (50%)	16 (59%)	14 (52%)	12 (55%)	12 (55%)
Years of experience as a CNE						
<1	6 (16%)	6 (27%)	6 (22%)	7 (26%)	4 (18%)	6 (27%)
1–2	6 (16%)	5 (23%)	6 (22%)	6 (22%)	4 (18%)	2 (9%)
3–4	10 (27%)	5 (23%)	8 (30%)	6 (22%)	5 (23%)	5 (23%)
5–6	5 (14%)	3 (14%)	3 (11%)	2 (7%)	4 (18%)	4 (18%)
7–8	3 (8%)	1 (5%)	1 (4%)	2 (7%)	2 (9%)	3 (14%)
9–10	3 (8%)	2 (9%)	2 (7%)	2 (7%)	1 (5%)	1 (5%)
11–12	3 (8%)	0 (0%)	0 (0%)	0 (0%)	1 (5%)	0 (0%)
13–14	1 (3%)	0 (0%)	1 (4%)	1 (4%)	1 (5%)	1 (5%)
≥15	0 (0%)	0 (0%)	0 (0%)	1 (4%)	0 (0%)	0 (0%)
Primary Clinical Area						
Critical care	6 (16%)	5 (23%)	6 (22%)	6 (22%)	4 (18%)	4 (18%)
Emergency department	1 (3%)	0 (0%)	1 (4%)	1 (4%)	1 (5%)	0 (0%)
Intermediate care	3 (8%)	2 (9%)	2 (7%)	2 (7%)	2 (9%)	2 (9%)
Medical surgical	14 (38%)	10 (45%)	8 (30%)	9 (33%)	7 (32%)	9 (41%)

Perinatal	3 (8%)	2 (9%)	5 (19%)	4 (15%)	4 (18%)	4 (18%)
Perioperative	3 (8%)	1 (5%)	2 (7%)	0 (0%)	1 (5%)	2 (9%)
Other	7 (19%)	2 (9%)	3 (11%)	5 (19%)	3 (14%)	1 (5%)
Highest nursing degree						
Associate's degree	2 (5%)	0 (0%)	0 (0%)	0 (0%)	0 (0%)	0 (0%)
Bachelor's degree	23 (62%)	17 (77%)	19 (70%)	18 (67%)	16 (73%)	14 (64%)
Master's degree	11 (30%)	5 (23%)	8 (30%)	9 (33%)	6 (27%)	8 (36%)
Doctoral degree	1 (3%)	0 (0%)	0 (0%)	0 (0%)	0 (0%)	0 (0%)

Table 2
Differences in responses pre versus post educational intervention

	Strongly Disagree	Somewhat Disagree	Neither Agree nor Disagree	Somewhat and Strongly Agree	P Value
I am comfortable initiating difficult conversations with my peers on the unit					
Needs assessment (n = 37)	1 (3%)	10 (27%)	8 (22%)	18 (49%)	<.01
Session 1 (n = 22)	0 (0%)	0 (0%)	2 (9%)	20 (91%)	
I am comfortable managing conflict within my professional environment					
Needs assessment (n = 37)	1 (3%)	7 (19%)	8 (22%)	21 (57%)	<.01
Session 2 (n = 22)	0 (0%)	0 (0%)	3 (14%)	19 (87%)	
I feel comfortable providing constructive feedback to new nurses on my unit					
Needs assessment (n = 37)	0 (0%)	1 (3%)	1 (3%)	35 (94%)	.89
Session 2 (n = 27)	0 (0%)	1 (4%)	0 (0%)	26 (96%)	
I feel comfortable providing constructive feedback to experienced nurses on my unit					
Needs assessment (n = 37)	0 (0%)	5 (14%)	2 (5%)	30 (81%)	.64
Session 2 (n = 27)	0 (0%)	5 (19%)	1 (4%)	20 (74%)	
It is important to debrief after stressful events in my practice area					
Debrief pre-survey (n = 27)	2 (7%)	0 (0%)	0 (0%)	24 (89%)	.49
Session 3 (n = 22)	0 (0%)	0 (0%)	0 (0%)	22 (100%)	
I am comfortable initiating a debrief after a stressful event in my practice area					
Debrief pre-survey (n = 27)	0 (0%)	6 (22%)	3 (11%)	17 (63%)	<.01
Session 3 (n = 22)	0 (0%)	0 (0%)	0 (0%)	22 (100%)	
Debriefing a non-critical event or simulation is important					
Debrief pre-survey (n = 27)	1 (4%)	1 (4%)	4 (15%)	20 (74%)	.06
Session 3 (n = 22)	0 (0%)	0 (0%)	1 (5%)	21 (96%)	
I am comfortable debriefing a non-critical event or simulation experience					
Debrief pre-survey (n = 27)	0 (0%)	5 (19%)	3 (11%)	18 (67%)	.11
Session 3 (n = 22)	0 (0%)	0 (0%)	1 (5%)	21 (95%)	
I am familiar with available resources to support staff with managing the effects of exposure to stressful events at the medical center					
Debrief pre-survey (n = 27)	1 (4%)	8 (30%)	5 (19%)	12 (45%)	<.01
Session 3 (n = 22)	0 (0%)	0 (0%)	0 (0%)	22 (100%)	
I have adequate opportunity to connect with my CNE colleagues					
Needs assessment	2 (5%)	11 (30%)	5 (14%)	19 (51%)	.19
Series evaluation	1 (5%)	1 (5%)	3 (14%)	16 (73%)	
I feel I am a valued member of the nursing leadership team on my unit					
Needs assessment	0 (0%)	3 (8%)	2 (5%)	32 (86%)	.63
Series evaluation	0 (0%)	3 (14%)	2 (9%)	18 (73%)	
I feel I am a valued member of the nursing leadership team at the medical center					
Needs assessment	2 (5%)	9 (24%)	4 (11%)	22 (59%)	.73
Series evaluation	1 (5%)	2 (9%)	3 (14%)	15 (68%)	

(continued on next page)

Table 2 (*continued*)					
	Strongly Disagree	**Somewhat Disagree**	**Neither Agree nor Disagree**	**Somewhat and Strongly Agree**	**P Value**
I have strong collegial relationships with my CNE colleagues					
Needs assessment	0 (0%)	6 (16%)	6 (16%)	25 (68%)	.48
Series evaluation	1 (5%)	2 (9%)	4 (18%)	14 (64%)	
I attend CNE workgroup meetings regularly					
Needs assessment	5 (14%)	3 (8%)	7 (19%)	22 (60%)	.07
Series evaluation	1 (5%)	4 (18%)	2 (9%)	14 (63%)	

It was helpful to hear the similarities between all the CNEs of what the work experience has been as we move into this role and then as we progress in this role. Interpersonal relationships certainly change once we became the CNE for the unit.

The challenge of difficult conversations

Clinical nurse educators described giving constructive feedback to more experienced staff and to staff with strong personalities as challenging. Clinical nurse educators described this challenge as related to their comfort level with initiating difficult conversations and the desire to deliver feedback in a thoughtful and non-punitive manner.

To have different, effective approaches (to facilitate difficult conversations) and talk through how other CNEs have handled difficult conversations and provide feedback is really helpful. It was also good to just talk about why giving feedback and/or constructive criticism to peers and colleagues can be difficult and uncomfortable.

Strategies for difficult conversations

Clinical nurse educators noted that communication tools and techniques would increase their confidence and ability to facilitate difficult conversations.

Having some tools to use when giving and receiving feedback will be great for me. I often struggle with not knowing what or how to say something so now I have some guidance to follow when planning how to give someone feedback.

Practicing effective communication techniques during the sessions led to CNE participants sharing personal experiences and group discussions of how others had successfully navigated similar situations. Taking the time to plan and prepare for a difficult conversation was identified by several CNEs as a strategy to improve their confidence and credibility during difficult conversations.

I think it was helpful to discuss strategies for navigating difficult conversations. The group discussions allowed us to compare experiences that everyone could relate to, and talk through how to best handle each situation.

Professional practice development

Clinical nurse educators commented that the session content provided opportunity for reflection and led to new ways of thinking about the CNE role.

This series has not only given me many tools to improve my communication skills within my role of CNE, but also allowed me to reflect on past events and think about how I can improve my communication moving forward.

Participants also recognized that the lack of formal orientation program to support their transition to the CNE role contributes to feelings of role isolation and they universally endorsed the need for ongoing professional development dedicated to the CNE group.

We don't have any training or education prior to starting the CNE role, and having difficult conversations is a vital (a frequent) part of the job. This is something that can be a hard adjustment to the role. Having the opportunity to learn about how to strategically have these conversations and being able to discuss challenging situations with colleagues in the same role is very valuable.

DISCUSSION

Clinical nurse educators are key contributors to the onboarding, orientation, and continued professional development of clinical nurses on their units, but participants in this intervention confirmed in their evaluations that CNEs themselves are negatively impacted by a lack of a similar focused onboarding and continued opportunities for professional development. Sustained high attendance in the sessions throughout the summer season (84.4%, 90.6%, and 81.3% total enrollment in Sessions 1, 2, and 3, respectively) demonstrated participants' prioritization of this opportunity. Clinical nurse educators self-identified need and prioritization of focused skill acquisition and development is consistent with the literature.[5,7] Ongoing professional development focused on leadership, communication techniques, clinical reflection, and learning and teaching strategies contribute to success in the CNE role.[2]

Clinical nurse educators played a central and very demanding role in just-in-time training for staff and were often the face and voice of multiple practice changes throughout the initial coronavirus disease 2019 (COVID 19) surge. Discussions during the in person sessions revealed CNEs often felt they lacked the communication skills to navigate difficult conversations and manage negative feedback from staff in spite of the organization's implementation of standard communication tools to escalate issues and disseminate process or practice changes.[9] Participant post-session survey responses endorsed the need for developing critical conversation skills to manage these challenging interactions. The heightened stress of the experience served to reinforce the importance and relevance of the original topics identified; difficult conversations and giving and receiving feedback, and identified a new one, conducting an effective debrief.

Interestingly, CNEs reported high levels of comfort with difficult conversations and giving feedback on Likert based items on the needs assessment. However, in response to the question "What educational and skill building opportunities would be most beneficial to your continued growth in your role as a CNE?", many respondents seemed to contradict that by identifying the aforementioned topics as most beneficial to their professional development. This discrepancy in CNE responses between Likert scale and open-ended questions may be related to acquiring new knowledge and methods for approaching difficult conversations introduced during the sessions and in interactive discussions with their peers. Discussions during live sessions, as well as in responses to open-ended evaluation questions confirmed that the education on communications related topics was exceedingly relevant and important to the professional development of CNEs. Balancing competing priorities of unit education and practice responsibilities, with director and organizational needs, likely impact the time available for CNEs' personal and professional development.[10] Responses seeking additional education about managing difficult conversations may be a response to wanting additional information on the topic or a desire for more professional development opportunities dedicated solely to CNEs.

There were improvements in CNEs' comfort with initiating difficult conversations with peers on their unit and with managing conflict in their professional environment on the Session 1 post-survey. Content from this session highlighted the value of addressing conflict to improve professional relationships and unit culture. Reviewing best practices for facilitating a difficult conversation and discussing strategies for successful outcomes allowed the participants to recognize that conversation skills require planning and practice. In session conversations allowed CNEs to realize that many of their peers also had feelings of anxiety related to initiating difficult conversations. These discussions led to participant responses of feeling less isolated in their role and able to reach out to a peer for support.

Before and after Session 2, CNEs reported more comfort in providing feedback to new nurses than to their experienced peers. During these sessions, CNEs expressed that providing feedback to new nurses was comfortable as their role was integral to the orientation of new nurses. Clinical nurse educators shared their experience giving feedback to experienced nurses as being more difficult and a contributor to role stress. Discussions revealed CNEs were more likely to be challenged on their knowledge or have their feedback be disregarded by more experienced nurses, which contributed to feelings of strain in their role. These examples of workplace incivility are well documented in nursing, although not specifically related to the CNE role, and reinforce the need for formal orientation, which includes strategies for approaching difficult conversations.[11] Clinical nurse educators also expressed difficulty with providing feedback to peers who continued to view them as their bedside colleague and not as a member of unit leadership. Assisting CNEs with overcoming interpersonal challenges related to role transition requires further exploration.

Clinical nurse educators were knowledgeable about debriefing after a critical event in their practice area but were less familiar with debriefing clinical situations as a method to develop staff critical thinking and reflective practice. After Session 3, statistically significant improvement was noted with participants feeling more comfortable initiating debrief after a stressful event and with increased knowledge about available resources to support staff with managing the effects of exposure to stressful events. In post-session survey responses, CNEs noted feeling more empowered to initiate a staff debrief after a stressful event on the unit, and to utilize debriefs in non-critical clinical situations to support the development of nurses critical thinking skills and reflective practice.

While robust participation in the online community was anticipated, there were only 9 participant-initiated posts over the course of the intervention. Forum posts detailed the application of communication strategies to challenging interactions in their professional practice. While these posts celebrated successful outcomes of difficult conversations, there was little interaction between participants in the online forum. As this was not a requirement for participation in the QI project, motivation to participate in the online forum may have been impacted by the participant's work or personal obligations.[12] Screen fatigue caused by COVID-19 related transitioning of all work-related meetings online may have also been a factor. Participants also expressed concerns related to the privacy of posts within the community, which may have contributed to lower rates of participation.

LIMITATIONS AND STRENGTHS

This QI project has several limitations. First, generalizability of findings is limited as the participants were recruited as convenience sample from a single medical center. The lack of a standard role definition further complicates generalizability of findings between organizations. Additionally, the CNEs who attended these sessions were self-selected and potentially more motivated than their counterparts who opted not to participate. Plans are underway to integrate findings from these sessions into a targeted transition to practice program to onboard all novice CNEs, thus controlling for self-selection bias in the future.

Another limitation to this QI project was the use of self-report as a measure of skills acquisition. An alternate method, such as real time peer observation and feedback, should be considered to evaluate the success of future series iterations. Finally, the QI project design did not include long-term follow-up with participants. Future work would benefit from evaluation of educational impact on participants' professional practice at 6- and 12-month intervals.

Initially, this intervention was designed as a large group session. Social distancing requirements within the institution restricted attendance to 10 people, including facilitators, to each session, which resulted in each session repeating 4 times per topic. Ultimately, participants cited the small group size as strength of the intervention in all of the session evaluations. Smaller sessions were less intimidating and invited open dialogue while promoting personal connections between CNEs.

SUMMARY/IMPLICATIONS FOR FUTURE CNE PROFESSIONAL DEVELOPMENT

This program revealed challenges that CNEs encountered, related to the absence of a formal orientation, to support their transition to the role. Without education regarding essential communication skills, CNEs expressed feeling stressed, isolated, and anxious when faced with initiating critical conversations. Clinical nurses transitioning into the CNE role will benefit from the development and implementation of a formal orientation supported by a mentor to assist with navigating their role transition.

CLINICS CARE POINTS

- Consider incorporating leadership and communication skills into CNE orientation to support transition to the role.
- Providing CNE specific professional development programs enhances networking and mentoring opportunities which may decrease feelings of role isolation and stress.

DISCLOSURE

The authors have no conflicts of interest to disclose.

REFERENCES

1. Callicutt D, Walker M. ANPD's revised scope and standards. J Nurses Prof Dev 2022;38(6):373–4.
2. Sayers J, DiGiacomo M, Davidson P. The nurse educator role in the acute care setting in Australia: important but poorly described. Aust J Adv Nurs 2011;28(4):44–52.
3. Fritz E. Transition from clinical to educator roles in nursing: an integrative review. J Nurses Prof Dev 2018;34(2):67–77.
4. Forbes VJ, Jessup AL. From expert to novice: the unnerving transition from experienced RN to neophyte APN. J Holist Nurs 2004;22(2):180–5.
5. Manning L, Neville S. Work-role transition: from staff nurse to clinical nurse educator. Nurs Prax N Z 2009;25(2):41–53.
6. McKinley MG. Go to the head of the class: clinical educator role transition. AACN Adv Crit Care 2009;20(1):91–101.

7. Coates K, Fraser K. A case for collaborative networks for clinical nurse educators. Nurse Educ Today 2014;34(1):6–10.

8. Harris P, Taylor R, Thielke R, et al. Research electronic data capture (REDCap) – a metadata-driven methodology and workflow process for providing translational research informatics support. J Biomed Inform 2009;42(2):377–81.

9. Sulmonte K, Bourie P, Carnevale K, et al. Flexibility in a crisis: how strong relational coordination and lean literacy helped us weather the COVID storm. Nurs Adm Q 2022;46(4):316–23.

10. Coffey J, White B. The clinical nurse educator role: a snapshot in time. J Contin Educ Nurs 2019;50(5):228–32.

11. Major K, Abderrahman E, Sweeney J. 'Crucial conversations' in the workplace. Am J Nurs 2013;114(4):66–70.

12. Nelson M, Oden K, Williams L. Student motivation to participate in asynchronous online discussions. J Nurs Educ Pract 2019;9(9):6–11.

Right-sizing Documentation
What the Pandemic Taught Us about Clinical Documentation and Quality of Care

Tiffany Kelley, PhD, MBA, RN, NI-BC, FNAP[a,b,c,*]

KEYWORDS

- Nursing documentation • COVID-19 • Nursing • Quality of care

KEY POINTS

- This article explores the available evidence of how nursing documentation contributed toward the delivery of quality care during the COVID-19 pandemic.
- Quality of care is grounded in 6 factors: safety, timeliness, equity, patient-centeredness, efficiency, and effectiveness.
- Nursing documentation continues to be an area of opportunity for the nursing profession to provide greater visibility into the profession's practice and impact on patient care.

INTRODUCTION

Nursing documentation is an essential component to the delivery of quality patient care.[1] Nursing documentation provides a method of collecting and communicating essential data, information, knowledge, and wisdom about a patient's care needs.[1] Nurses and all other health care professionals need accurate and available access to patient's health information to make timely and informed patient care decisions.[1] On March 11, 2020, the United States was faced with the start of a global pandemic.[2] Coronavirus (eg, COVID-19) was the first global pandemic of its magnitude in 100 years,[3] and the first time nurses were faced with an enduring emergency of that magnitude.[4] At the start of the pandemic, nurses (*as well as the public*) had limited knowledge of how COVID-19 spread to patients and how to effectively treat patients.[5] However, nurses did have the ability to communicate patients' clinical and personal health status to maintain the individuality of each patient through nursing documentation. The purpose of this review is to explore the available evidence of how nursing documentation contributed toward the delivery of quality care during the COVID-19 pandemic.

---

[a] Healthcare Innovation Online Graduate Certificate Program, Nursing and Engineering Innovation Center, University of Connecticut, School of Nursing, Storrs, CT, USA; [b] iCare Nursing Solutions, Boston, MA, USA; [c] Nightingale Apps, Boston, MA, USA
* Corresponding author.
E-mail address: tiffany.kelley@uconn.edu

Crit Care Nurs Clin N Am 36 (2024) 393–406
https://doi.org/10.1016/j.cnc.2024.04.001
0899-5885/24/© 2024 Elsevier Inc. All rights reserved.

BACKGROUND

Nurses continue to represent the largest group of health care professionals with 27 million nurses worldwide,[6] approximately 6 million in North America and 5.2 million in the United States.[7] Nurses are the largest group of health care professionals in acute and critical care hospital settings. Nurses collect up to 50% of the data and information needed for care delivery, more than any other single member of the health care team.[8] Since 2019, before the global COVID-19 pandemic, 96% of hospitals in the United States used electronic health records (EHRs) to collect and communicate patient health information.[9] Electronic nursing documentation and other EHR components were expected to further advance health care quality.[10,11] Yet, the current state of nursing documentation has opportunities for improvement in addressing the unique characteristics of the patient,[12,13] nurses' unique contributions to health care,[14] and overall ability to interact with the electronic nursing documentation in a way that supports efficient and effective nursing workflows to deliver quality patient care.[1]

Quality of Care

The Institute of Medicine[11] defined quality according to 6 factors in Crossing the Quality Chasm. Those 6 factors include that care is safe, effective, efficient, equitable, timely, and patient-centered.[11] Safe care is the ability to prevent unintended injury or harm.[11] Effective care is care provided based on current available evidence to avoid overuse, underuse, or misuse of potential treatments.[11] Efficient care avoids unnecessary waste of time, services, treatments, and more.[11] Equitable care is the provision of care that accounts for social determinants of health (SDoH) in how care is provided to meet the patient's optimal health status.[11] Timely care is the removal of potential delays or waiting in care delivery.[11] Last, patient-centered care is care that acknowledges and integrates individual care preferences and needs into the care plan.[11] Each of these factors has an influence on the ability for nurses to deliver quality patient care. Nursing documentation has a role in supporting nurses' ability to provide quality care across all 6 of these factors.

Nursing Documentation

Nursing documentation is a tool for collecting and communicating clinical patient information essential to make informed and knowledgeable decisions for quality care. Nursing documentation is a component of an EHR.[15] With at least 96% of hospitals and health centers using EHRs,[9] nurses are primarily using electronic-based documentation intended, in part, to support care based on the patient's needs and health status. Such electronic nursing documentation systems must meet regulatory requirements. However, not all the essential clinical and personal information needed to know their patients[13] for quality care are based on those regulatory requirements. Thus, nurses are often documenting for regulatory requirements in addition to communicating with caregivers about the patient's clinical and personal health information needed for optimal quality care delivery. The documentation needs can also vary depending on clinical care areas.[1] The unexpectedness and lack of knowledge during the COVID-19 pandemic required nurses and other members of the health care team to have as much information about their patients as possible, placing even more dependency and urgency on nurses' documentation.

Coronavirus Pandemic and Nurses

The COVID-19 global pandemic occurred during the Year of the Nurse.[14] The Year of the Nurse marked the 200th anniversary of Florence Nightingale's birthday.[15]

Nightingale was one of the original nursing pioneers. She advocated for preventative measures in health care such as clean air and water in her report, "Notes on Nursing."[16] Nightingale also recognized the power of each nurse's contribution to the patient's needs through documentation, "learn to ask for and appreciate the information of a nurse, who is at once a careful observer and a clear reporter."[16] To be a "clear reporter" today, can be translated to mean an effective communicator through verbal, written, and electronic communication tools. While nurses know how to care for patients with familiar illnesses, the coronavirus pandemic introduced a new virus. Very few, if any, nurses were fully prepared in how to effectively treat the highly infectious virus when it began to infect patients in the United States. As a result, nurses' ability to effectively communicate with each other as well as about their patients was of great importance during this time. Nursing documentation is the available tool to support the necessary information and knowledge needs across the care team.

METHODS

A database search of PubMed and the Cumulative Index for Nursing and Allied Health Literature was first conducted using the key terms "nursing documentation" and "COVID-19." Both terms were required to be in the title or abstract. The search resulted in a total of 7 articles for review. After a manual review of the 7 articles, 3 were included in the review. A second search of PubMed was conducted using the terms documentation and nursing and COVID-19. All 3 terms were required to be in the title or abstract with full text available and in English. This search returned 36 articles, 5 articles were duplicates from the first search. Other excluded articles did not specifically include nursing documentation in the research or quality improvement projects. Manual review of the titles of those 36 articles led to the inclusion of a total of 6 additional articles. This article includes a review of 9 articles.

RESULTS

The author reviewed the 9 articles in context of the 6 factors of health care quality. The 6 factors are grouped into 3 sections for analysis: *safe and timely care*, *equity and patient-centered care*, and *efficient and effective care* (**Table 1**). Each of the 9 articles represents at least one of the 6 factors of health care quality. The results will describe how the new knowledge during the pandemic contributes to quality care through nursing documentation in the context of these factors of quality.

Safe and Timely Care

To deliver safe care is to prevent any unintended harm or injury to patients.[11] To deliver timely care is to reduce wait times and delays for those in need of care.[11] Personal protective equipment (PPE) was of great importance and need during the pandemic. PPE includes gloves, masks, and gowns donned by nurses and health care professionals to protect nurses and health care professionals from spreading viruses and organisms to other humans. PPE was in extreme demand while faced with extreme shortages during the COVID-19 pandemic. Thus, in a retrospective chart review, Albright and colleagues[17] sought out to investigate the effectiveness of the Emerging Infectious Disease Surveillance Tool (EMD) to screen for the presence of COVID-19 for patients in advance of being admitted to a hospital (see **Table 1**). The study evaluated at total of 13,399, emergency 911 calls made from March 8 to July 2020, to evaluate patients at high risk for COVID-19 through a series of short questions with responses of "Y" or "N."[17] The EMD screening tool was only able to accurately detect COVID-19-positive patients 25% of the time.[17] While intended to provide a timely information

Table 1
Review of articles

Reference	Purpose	Design	Sample	Instrument	Key Findings	Discussion
Safe and Timely Care						
Albright et al,[17] 2021	To determine the efficacy of a previously developed screening tool aiming to identify patients who test + for COVID-19 on the appropriate use of PPE.	Retrospective chart review	Collection of 911 calls between March 8, 2020 and July 31, 2020.	Emerging Infectious Disease (EMD) Surveillance Tool	Of 13,399 calls, 4329 patients screened positive for COVID-19 with the EMD. A total of 263 had a positive COVID-19 test. Of that 263, 74.9% also had a positive EMD screen.	Further investigation is recommended to identify greater sensitivity of the tool and/or adjustments to the screening questions. Such a documentation tool has continued value for screening high-risk patients in an effort to conserve and appropriately use PPE.
Patel et al,[18] 2022	To investigate the emergence of 7 CLABSIs during the 5 month period of November 2020 and March 2021 with no CLABSIs detected in the 18 mo before November 2020.	Retrospective chart review	Patients with a CLABSI at the VHA Nebraska-Western Iowa Health Care System	Date elements: Line insertion date Date of bacteremia detection Species and susceptibility of organism Location of the patient Health care provider who inserted the line	The investigation of the presence of a CLABSI in February 2021 revealed deviations in training, documentation, and practice protocols for nurses with regard to central line dressing changes. Inpatient	While changes in nursing documentation could have contributed to the presence of CLABSIs during this time, there are other potential influencing factors that also could have contributed.

	Purpose	Method	Sample	Framework/Analysis	Results	Conclusions
					MD and RN responsible for patient	documentation had been changed (eg, "streamlined") in March 2020 (eg, the start of the pandemic in the United States) with less detailed guidelines on central line dressing care.
Faulds et al,[19] 2021	To implement a continuous glucose monitoring (CGM) practice guideline for intravenous insulin administration with the goal of reducing point-of-care glucose monitoring checks during the COVID-19 pandemic.	Focus groups	A total of 9 nurses caring for COVID-19-positive patients on CGM in an MICU setting.	A priori code book developed from the semistructured focus group interview questions.	Four themes emerged: 1. Accuracy 2. Nursing ownership 3. Workflow 4. Barriers and suggestions	The use of CGM in ICU settings has great potential even beyond the pandemic to improve timeliness of care, support patient health outcomes and maximize the safety of the patients and providers in the event of a pandemic.

Equitable and Patient-centered Care

	Purpose	Method	Sample	Framework/Analysis	Results	Conclusions
Banister et al,[20] 2022	To explore the types and frequency of nurse-sensitive indicators identified in nursing documentation of adult patients during the COVID-19 pandemic.	Retrospective chart review	Analysis of 94 patient records.	Gordon's Eleven Functional Health Patterns (FHP) Framework as a guide to analyze clinical, social, and nursing assessment data elements.	Nine of 11 FHPs present in nurse-sensitive indicators. Inconsistent SDoH documentation.	Documentation gaps were identified that could impact ability to provide quality care.

(continued on next page)

Table 1
(continued)

Reference	Purpose	Design	Sample	Instrument	Key Findings	Discussion
Wagner et al,[21] 2022	To identify terminology gaps and opportunities for new nursing diagnoses (NANDA), interventions (NIC), and outcomes (NOC) and linkages to be used during a pandemic for nursing documentation.	Seven nurse experts formed consensus frameworks to develop NANDA, NIC, and NOC linkages.	NANDA-I existing diagnoses	Analysis of existing NANDA-I diagnosis labels and identified potential interventions (NIC) and outcomes (NOC)	Seven nursing diagnoses identified in 3 NANDA-I domains. Fifty-four different NIC interventions identified. Eighty-nine different NOC outcomes identified.	This analysis creates opportunities to provide more sensitive and specific documentation using terminologies during a pandemic.
Monsen et al,[22] 2021	To explore the concept of resilience in available nursing documentation datasets before and during the COVID-19 pandemic.	Retrospective correlation study	Three samples: (1) Pre-COVID-19 community-generated data (2) Pre-COVID-19 clinical documentation data (3) During COVID-19 community-generated data	The Omaha System	Resilience was detectable before and during the COVID-19 pandemic from the available data.	Standardized documentation allows for effective assessment across clinical care areas. Resilience is a concept in need of inclusion in documentation.
Balice-Bourgois et al,[23] 2022	To explore the (1) needs of COVID-19 patients; (2) the nursing interventions and outcomes; and (3) the experiences of nurses, patients and caregivers.	Mixed-method convergent study design	Nurses Patients Caregivers	The study will consist of 3 phases with questionnaires, interviews, data collection and nursing documentation.	This study discussed the development of the study protocol to be used in a future study.	

Efficient and Effective Care

Holub et al,[24] 2023	Quality improvement project	This quality improvement project sought to optimize and streamline documentation.	Memorial Hermann Health System (MHHS) in Houston, Texas (17 acute care hospitals).	Cyclical model for managing change with a clinically led electronic medical record optimization (CLEO) team	Direct care nurses redesigned EMR bands that led to 20% reduction in data elements within each assessment. Improved user experience for nurses.	The CLEO team has additional plans to make improvements but will prioritize based on survey feedback.
Livesay et al,[25] 2023	Qualitative interviews	To explore sociotechnical challenges nurse encounter when using digital health tools during the pandemic.	16 nurses consisting of 5 groups	Semistructured interview protocol	Analysis of interviews revealed these themes: 1. Technical challenges 2. Nurse–technology interaction 3. Content management 4. Training/human resources 5. Communication and workflow 6. Internal policies and guidelines 7. External factors 8. Effectiveness assessment for postpandemic use and integration	Nurse involvement across roles is important in order to support the effective use and sociotechnical deployment of digital health tools.

Abbreviations: MD, medical doctor; MICU, medical intensive care unit; RN, registered nurse.

source, there remains risk for inaccurate detection.[17] The investigators noted the need to continue to use clinical judgment in tandem with the dispatch screening tool for the presence of COVID-19.[17] While the EMD tool was able to successfully identify a patient positive for COVID-19, 25% of the time, there remains opportunity for additional refinement of the instrument's sensitivity to detect COVID-19. The clinical impact could lead to greater accuracy in determining whether PPE is or is not needed for a patient. Accuracy of PPE usage has the potential to increase the safety of the directly and indirectly affected patients, nurses, and health care professionals.

Central line-associated bloodstream infections (CLABSIs) are hospital-acquired infections. The Veterans Health Administration (VHA) Nebraska-Western Iowa Health Care System had no reported CLABSIs for 18 months between April 2019 and November 2020.[18] However, the investigators reported at least one CLABSI per month for a total of 7 over a 5 month period between November 2020 and March 2021 during the pandemic (see **Table 1**).[18] The investigators noted that the electronic nursing documentation had been streamlined in March 2020 in preparation for a new EHR.[18] The investigators noted that the changes to documentation alongside educational training changes on how to document central line dressing changes could have contributed to unintended consequences to central line care.[18] CLABSIs are preventable and were prevented for 18 months at this facility before November 2020.[18] While it is not known the extent to which nursing documentation could have contributed to the presence of CLABSIs during that time frame, there remains opportunity to improve documentation to strive for the safest possible patient care. CLABSIs are one area where further investigation can occur on the relationship between nursing documentation and an unfavorable patient outcome.

The presence of COVID-19 in hospitalized patients posed a safety and timeliness of care risk for poor glycemic control and potentially higher mortality rates.[19] A multidisciplinary team formed to investigate the potential for reducing point of care (POC) glucose monitoring as a mechanism to reduce health care worker exposure to COVID-19 (see **Table 1**).[19] As an alternative, the team developed a clinical guideline for the use of continuous glucose monitoring (CGM) for intensive care patients in need of intravenous insulin during the COVID-19 pandemic.[19] Through the development of a new protocol and interviews with a focus group of 9 nurses, the use of the CGM earned the trust of the CGMs values in place of POC monitoring. Nurses' exposure to COVID-19 was reduced. There was a desire to continue this protocol beyond the immediate need during the pandemic.[19] The investigators noted an opportunity to improve the EHR documentation with CGM to ensure consistency across caregivers.[19] Such a data element would require a new field in the EHR for consistent documentation.[19]

In the abovementioned 3 clinically oriented investigations that occurred during the COVID-19 pandemic, all leveraged nursing documentation in some capacity to evaluate care quality. While the premise of their investigations was not solely focused on nursing documentation, they required data and information from the documentation. There were many opportunities to improve safe and timely care during the pandemic. These 3 investigations each explored a different opportunity: (1) early identification of a positive COVID-19 test for safe and timely PPE use; (2) dressing change documentation to prevent the presence of CLABSIs, a safety risk for patients; and (3) the use of CGM to provide timely care while safely reducing nurses' exposure to COVID-19.

Equitable and Patient-centered Care

Equitable care delivery should not vary due to a person's characteristics (eg, *gender, race, economic status*) or SDoH.[11] Patient-centered care delivery is related to equitable care.[11] Patient-centered care is delivered with respect and responsiveness to an individual patient's specific care preferences.[11] Measuring patient centered care through nursing documentation can be approached in a variety of ways, including nurse-sensitive indicators. Banister and colleagues explored nurse-sensitive indicators in relation to the clinical and sociodemographic characteristics of admitted coronavirus patients during the initial surge of COVID-19 in 2020 (see **Table 1**).[20] A total of 94 patients' charts were reviewed for demographic data, clinical information, and health outcomes.[20] The investigators detected that data and information needed to immediately care for COVID-19 patients were adequately documented in the EHRs.[20] However, there was a gap in biopsychosocial health and SDoH data.[20] Such data are noted by the investigators to aid in ensuring the ability to provide holistic and equitable patient care.[20]

Patient-centered care often extends beyond the individual patient to include the patients' family who often aide in delivery of care. Nurses use the nursing process to assess patients and their needs. The nursing process includes identifying appropriate nursing diagnoses, interventions to address those diagnoses and associated outcomes. North American Nursing Diagnosis Association (NANDA), Nursing Interventions Classification (NIC), and Nursing Outcomes Classification (NOC) are 3 ANA-recognized standardized nursing terminologies that were used in Wagner and colleagues to identify potential documentation gaps in family-related components of patient care.[21] COVID-19 presented unique challenges for patient and family care (see **Table 1**).[21] Through an evaluation of existing North American Nursing Diagnosis Association International (NANDA-I) diagnoses, the investigators identified 7 NANDA-I nursing diagnoses to use in order to link nursing interventions and outcomes for documentation. The nursing diagnoses aligned with one of 3 NANDA-I domains. The 3 identified domains are (1) health promotion, (2) role relationship, and (3) coping/stress tolerance. Additionally, a total of 15 new terminologies were identified as needed to support nursing documentation in a pandemic situation. Of those 15 terminologies, a total of 5 nursing diagnoses (eg, NANDA), 3 nursing interventions (eg, NIC), and 7 nursing outcomes (eg, NOC) were identified as opportunities for additional documentation terminology needs to include as options for nurses to use to describe their care delivery associated with the family response needs during a pandemic.[21] In a digital documentation environment with great dependency on structured data elements such as drop downs and pick lists, having predetermined options allows for consistency of care delivery as well as more appropriate selection of terms to describe the patient's individualized care needs. Additionally, the use of structured nursing recognized terminologies allows for advancement in effective aggregation of data and potential ease of any interoperable data exchange needs in the future.

Another layer of person-centered care explored during the COVID-19 pandemic was the concept of resilience. Resilience is the ability to withstand and adapt to difficulties and challenges in life experiences. The COVID-19 pandemic was new for everyone. Resilience was essential for all during the COVID-19 pandemic.[22] However, those in need of nursing care were even more vulnerable to changes in their resilience. Monsen and colleagues analyzed datasets to explore whole person health at the individual and population level.[22] As part of this effort, the investigators sought out to explore the necessary documentation to capture resilience as part of whole person health.[22] The Omaha System was the ANA-recognized standardized nursing terminology utilized as part of this evaluation.[22] While the researchers were able to confirm that whole person health, including resilience, can be captured through the Omaha System, there is room for improvement in the volume and quality of data contributed to the patient's health record.[22] Standardized nursing terminologies such as the Omaha System and NANDA, NIC, and NOC are necessary for our profession to be able to communicate consistent concepts across systems.

Balice-Bourgois and colleagues also sought out to explore aspects of patient-centered care in the context of a study protocol to evaluate patients' experiences and needs during the pandemic (see **Table 1**).[23] The investigators created the protocol to explore nursing care delivery and associated patient care needs across one's hospital inpatient stay.[23] When executed, data will be collected using Cantarelli's Nursing Performance Model of 11 categories of fundamental nursing needs.[23] These nursing needs include breathing, safe environment, interacting, and communication and 8 other categories. From this study protocol, the team aims to explore where patients benefit from specific nursing care interventions during their illnesses.[23] This presents the opportunity to identify potential gaps in equitable and patient-centeredness of care. Additionally, the findings will offer insights into how to document care needs for patients with COVID-19 during their illness.[23] The ability to leverage nursing documentation to communicate across the health team is limited without a mechanism to document care needs specific to an illness.

Efficient and Effective Care

To deliver efficient care is to eliminate waste.[11] Effective care delivery relies on evidence-based practice guidelines and protocols.[11] Quality care delivery relies on both efficiency and effectiveness from the nurses delivering care. Documentation burden is a known professional issue in nursing and health care. During the surge of COVID-19, Holub and Giergerich embarked on a quality improvement project in an effort to reduce the nurses' documentation burden (see **Table 1**).[24] This team developed a clinically led electronic medical record optimization (CLEO) approach to reduce nurses' documentation requirements.[24] The CLEO team was able to enable clinicians to lead change through the redesign of EHR assessments.[24] The changes resulted in at least a 20% reduction in required data elements.[24] Nurses recognized the changes as contributing toward higher usability of the EHR.[24] The team anticipates additional phases of CLEO beyond the COVID-19 surge to work to continued efforts at alleviating nursing documentation burden.[24]

Beyond the fields to document, nurses need to be able to effectively use the digital tools that are present to efficiently manage the data, information, knowledge, and wisdom needed about the patient for quality care. Integrating digital tools for nursing care delivery and documentation is complex with multiple contributing factors. Livesay and colleagues conducted an exploration of sociotechnical challenges during the pandemic around digital health tools took place through 16 interviews with 5 different groups of nurses.[25] Bedside nurses to Chief Nursing Information Officers expressed a total of 8 categories of sociotechnical challenges. These challenges included the technical capabilities of digital tools, training of the new digital tools, external factors such as regulations, internal organizational cultural processes, and nurses' interactions with the digital tools.[25] Delivery of efficient and effective care does depend on one's ability to use the available digital tools.[25] The investigators recommend increasing nurse involvement in the system design life cycle of new digital tools. With the identified categories in this exploratory study, additional research is recommended to explore the sociotechnical factors that influence nurses' ability to efficiently and effectively use digital tools for care delivery.[25]

DISCUSSION

This article sought out to explore the available evidence of how nursing documentation contributed toward the delivery of quality care during the COVID-19 pandemic. A total of 9 peer review articles were identified for review. The articles were organized and evaluated to identify the implications on care quality. Each article approached the role of nursing documentation during the COVID-19 pandemic in different ways. However, there were some consistencies across the articles, regardless of the evaluated care concept(s). First, there remains opportunity for improvement in how nursing documentation is used as a formal artifact of provided care. Second, there is interest in leveraging nursing documentation to support care needs in the moment. However, there remain sociotechnical challenges that prevent full knowledge integration with nurses in the present moment as well as historical retrospective reviews of nursing documentation datasets. This suggests that to continue to right-size documentation for optimal quality care delivery, nurses need the financial, technical, and organizational culture support to approach nursing documentation as that primary source to communicate patients' health needs and serve as a document of record for patients and population-level evaluations.

Limitations

The author wrote this article in the Fall of 2023. The World Health Organization declared a global pandemic of COVID-19 on March 11, 2020.[2] There was a limited body of published, peer-reviewed evidence to explore how nursing documentation contributed toward the delivery of quality care during the COVID-19 pandemic. Owing to the level of emergency, need for nurses to provide direct care and severity of illness, it is likely that hospitals and health centers were making rapid documentation changes to address information needs but were not yet able to publish such research and quality improvement projects. One way to address this limitation is to encourage publication of any research or quality improvement efforts to offer insights for how to continue to deliver quality care through nursing documentation.

Implications for Practice

Nursing documentation is a core component of nursing care delivery. Historically, nurses have had the perspective of, "*if it is not documented, then it is not done.*" This statement is often conditioned early in one's nursing practice. What is missing from this perspective is the recognition of the value that nursing documentation brings as a communication tool about the patient's status and needs. In the analyzed articles, nursing documentation was referenced as a source to measure aspects of quality care delivery. However, in many instances, the documentation was not sufficient to serve as the sole tool for data and information to evaluate care quality. The identified gaps and/or unknowns as a result of retrospective reviews indicate that we continue to have room for improvement in how we view nursing documentation's role in nursing and how we can shift toward a perspective of appreciating documentation as a visible source for the actions and efforts of nurses to provide safe, effective, efficient, equitable, timely, and patient-centered care.

Implications for Research and Innovation

The available literature that evaluated elements of nursing documentation for care quality was limited in scope. However, what is known is that more research and discovery is needed to identify how to reinforce the role of nursing documentation in a proactive way. Rather than reducing nursing documentation to an action that is either "done" or "not done," the nursing profession must emphasize and demonstrate the value of documentation for our ability to provide high-quality care over time. Additionally, proactive or prospective research studies that explore how nursing documentation is (or is not) used in the day-to-day care delivery would reveal opportunities for new advancements in technology, processes, and/or other gaps that retrospective chart review studies cannot reveal. As health care continues to become more digitally dependent, nursing must continue to identify ways to effectively integrate documentation sources and tools into care delivery for the benefit of the patient's immediate and future care needs.

SUMMARY

This review of the literature explored the available evidence of how nursing documentation contributed toward the delivery of quality care during the COVID-19 pandemic. The available literature sought to evaluate different aspects of care quality through available nursing documentation data. Yet, their findings collectively reveal that there remain continued opportunities to reinforce the value and importance of documentation whether in a pandemic or not. The nursing profession must continue to integrate documentation sources and tools into care delivery for the patient's individual record as well as a collective aggregate record for population-level data evaluation over time.

CLINICS CARE POINTS

- Nursing documentation is recognized as a tool that is necessary to communicate patient care needs for quality care.
- Nursing documentation was leveraged as a tool during the coronavirus pandemic to evaluate actions taken to provide safe, timely, equitable, patient-centered, efficient, and effective care.
- As a profession, nursing must recognize the long-term impact of nursing documentation for quality care delivery and find ways to ensure more complete documentation across all areas of necessary clinical and personal patient information.
- The very limited number of studies that explored the role of nursing documentation in aiding aspects of quality care during the COVID-19 pandemic may be reflective of the overwhelming nature of the day-to-day nursing and care delivery process during that time.
- To proactively support nurses in any future pandemic or critical care emergency, nurses must evaluate how to build workflow systems that support clinical and personal information needs for safe and timely care, equity and patient-centered care, and efficient and effective care.

DISCLOSURE

The author has nothing to disclose.

REFERENCES

1. Kelley T. Information use with paper and electronic nursing documentation by nurses caring for pediatric patients. Dissertation. Durham: Duke University; 2012.
2. World Health Organization. WHO Director-General's opening remarks at the media briefing on COVID-19 – 11 March 2020. Available at: https://www.who.int/director-general/speeches/detail/who-director-general-s-opening-remarks-at-the-media-briefing-on-covid-19—11-march-2020. [Accessed 1 November 2023].
3. Morens D, Taubenberger J, Fauci A. A centenary tale of two pandemics: the 1918 influenza pandemic and COVID-19, Part I. Am J Public Health 2021;111(6): 1086–94.

4. Chan G, Bitton J, Elliott D. The impact of COVID-19 on the nursing workforce: a national overview. OJIN 2021;26:2.
5. Alvarez E, Bielska I, Hopkins S, et al. Limitations of COVID-19 testing and case data for evidence-informed health policy and practice. Health Res Policy Sys 2023;21:11.
6. World Health Organization. Nursing and midwifery. Available at: https://www.who.int/news-room/fact-sheets/detail/nursing-and-midwifery. [Accessed 1 November 2023].
7. American Association of Colleges of Nursing. Nursing workforce fact sheet. Available at: https://www.aacnnursing.org/news-data/fact-sheets/nursing-workforce-fact-sheet. [Accessed 1 November 2023].
8. Kelley TF, Brandon D. Development of an observational tool to measure nurses' information needs. NI 2012;2012:209.
9. HealthIT.gov. National trends in hospital and physician adoption of electronic health records. Available at: https://www.healthit.gov/data/quickstats/national-trends-hospital-and-physician-adoption-electronic-health-records. [Accessed 1 November 2023].
10. Kohn KT, Corrigan JM, Donaldson MS, editors. Committee on quality health care in America. Washington, DC: Institute of Medicine: National Academy Press; 1999.
11. Institute of Medicine (US) Committee on Quality of Health Care in America. Crossing the quality Chasm: a new health system for the 21st Century. Washington, DC: National Academies Press (US); 2001.
12. Kelley TF, Brandon DH, Docherty SL. Electronic nursing documentation as a strategy to improve quality of patient care. J Nurs Scholarsh 2011;43(2):154–62.
13. Kelley T, Docherty S, Brandon D. Information needed to support knowing the patient. ANS Adv Nurs Sci 2013;36(4):351–63.
14. World Health Organization. Year of the nurse and Midwife 2020. Available at: https://www.who.int/campaigns/annual-theme/year-of-the-nurse-and-the-midwife-2020. [Accessed 28 November 2023].
15. Sherifali D. The Year of the nurse, Florence Nightingale and COVID-19: Reflections from social isolation. Can J Diabetes 2020;44(4):293–4.
16. Nightingale F. Notes on nursing. Garden City, NY: Dover Publications; 1969.
17. Albright A, Gross K, Hunter M, et al. A dispatch screening tool to identify patients at high risk for COVID-19 in the prehospital setting. West J Emerg Med 2021; 22(6):1253–6.
18. Patel S, Rajan A, Azeem A, et al. Outbreak of central-line-associated bloodstream infections (CLABSIs) amid the coronavirus disease 2019 (COVID-19) pandemic associated with changes in central-line dressing care accompanying changes in nursing education, nursing documentation, and dressing supply kits. Infect Control Hosp Epidemiol 2022;1:1–3.
19. Faulds E, Jones L, McNett M, et al. Facilitators and barriers to nursing implementation of continuous glucose monitoring (CGM) in critically ill patients with COVID-19. Endocr Pract 2021;27(4):354–61.
20. Banister G, Carroll D, Dickins K, et al. Nurse-sensitive indicators during COVID-19. Int J Nurs Knowl 2022;33:234–44.
21. Wagner C, Swanson E, Moorhead S, et al. NANDA-I, NOC, and NIC linkages to SARS-CoV-2 (COVID-19): Part 3. Family response. Int J Nurs Knowl 2022;33:5–17.
22. Monsen K, Austin R, Goparaju B, et al. Exploring large community- and clinically generated datasets to understand resilience before and during the COVID-19 pandemic. J Nurs Scholarsh 2021;53:262–9.

23. Balice-Bourgois C, Bonetti L, Tolotti A, et al. Experiences and needs of patients, caregivers and nurses during the COVID-19 pandemic: study protocol for a mixed-methods multicentre study. Int J Environ Res Public Health 2022;19:1–9.
24. Holub M, Giergerich C. Decreasing the nursing documentation burden during the Covid-19 surge. Nurse Lead 2023 Feb;21(1):38–41.
25. Livesay K, Petersen S, Walker, et al. Sociotechnical challenges of digital health in nursing practice during the COVID-19 pandemic: national study. JMIR Nurs 2023;6:e46819.

Health Equities with Limited English Proficiency
A Review of the Literature

Ashley L. O'Donoghue, PhD[a],*, Tenzin Dechen, MPH[a],
Sharon C. O'Donoghue, DNP, RN[b]

KEYWORDS

- Limited English proficiency • LEP • Language barrier • Health-care disparities
- Culturally competent care • Health-care delivery

KEY POINTS

- Health equity exists when everyone has an equal opportunity to achieve their highest level of health.
- Effective communication is not always established with patients with limited English proficiency (LEP).
- Communication barriers can lead to longer hospital stays, an increase in adverse events, and poorer outcomes.
- Federal regulation requires hospitals to provide medically trained interpreters; however, this does not always occur.
- These findings highlight the complex challenges that patients with LEP face in the health-care system and the crucial need for targeted interventions to enhance language access.

INTRODUCTION

Health equity exists when everyone has a fair, equal opportunity to achieve their highest level of health. To attain this, health-care organizations must overcome many obstacles to eliminate disparities.[1] Effective communication is essential to ensure a therapeutic, trusting relationship between the patient and health-care providers.[2] Unfortunately, effective communication is not always established with patients with limited English proficiency (LEP) and their families.

Patients with LEP are defined as those with limited capacity to speak, read, write, or understand English.[3] More than 25 million people in the United States have LEP, and

[a] Center for Healthcare Delivery Science, Beth Israel Deaconess Medical Center, 330 Brookline Avenue, Boston, MA 02215, USA; [b] Lois E. Silverman Department of Nursing, Beth Israel Deaconess Medical Center, 330 Brookline Avenue, Boston, MA 02215, USA
* Corresponding author.
E-mail address: aodonogh@bidmc.harvard.edu

Crit Care Nurs Clin N Am 36 (2024) 407–413
https://doi.org/10.1016/j.cnc.2024.01.004
0899-5885/24/© 2024 Elsevier Inc. All rights reserved.
ccnursing.theclinics.com

this number continues to increase.[4] Patients with LEP experience communication barriers that can lead to longer hospital stays, increased adverse events, and poorer outcomes.[5,6] Federal regulation requires hospitals to provide medically trained interpreters; however, this does not always occur.[7] Clinicians often cite difficulty in accessing an interpreter in a timely manner as the primary reason for not using one.[8] In the absence of a medically trained interpreter, clinicians may use a patient's family member or attempt to do their best to communicate without a shared common language. These attempts at communicating without a medically trained interpreter leave patients and their families disadvantaged. Effective communication is essential in critical care environments where understanding the diagnosis, treatment options, and care goals is imperative. The purpose of this article is to review and summarize the published literature on the care of critically ill patients with LEP and to identify areas for improvement. We identified 3 broad areas of current research: communication barriers, outcomes, and health-care costs.

COMMUNICATION BARRIERS

Effective communication in health care often breaks down for patients and families with LEP, resulting in suboptimal care experiences.[9–11] Although many health-care clinicians identify a lack of interpreters as a reason why one is not used; Diamond and colleagues[8] identified other variables. Resident physician described using family members to interpret for convenience and thought they could "get by," even though they believed patients with LEP were receiving suboptimal care. These challenges were further exacerbated by the coronavirus disease 2019 (COVID-19) pandemic, marked by interpreter shortages and social distancing measures.[12] The hospital landscape changed drastically during the pandemic. The availability of in-hospital interpreters decreased significantly due to the potential for the COVID-19 transmission,[9] and family visitations were restricted.[12] This restriction had a negative impact on patients with LEP because family members are often used to interpret for their loved ones. This negatively effected communication and decision-making in the intensive care units (ICUs).

Much literature on LEP and health communication in critical care environments revolves around end-of-life care decision-making. One study showed disparities among patients with LEP in the ICU because they were less likely to have critical orders or advance directives and are more likely to have prolonged mechanical ventilation and restraint use. In addition, interpreting concepts such as palliative care proved to be a common challenge for patients with LEP and their families.[13] Another study observed clinicians spent twice as much time communicating and offering support to English-speaking family members compared with patients with LEP and families, even in interpreted settings, which indicates the importance of requiring cultural openness for patients with LEP and families.[14]

Ju (2021) reports variations in the use of interpreter services by health-care provider type. Physicians and nurse practitioners were most likely to use interpreters, especially during detailed history taking and at discharge. However, the study reported lower interpreter use by registered nurses and lower use during care delivery, such as medication administration and procedures. Even when interpreter services were accessible, their utilization remained inconsistent throughout the patient encounter. For example, Spanish-speaking patients with LEP reported using interpreters at least once on average during their health-care encounters but the duration of interpreter use comprised only a third of overall interaction.[15] Thus, even institutions that capture data on whether or not an interpreter was used may lack nuance on when and how much an interpreter was used during a patient interaction.

Preventing errors and improving outcomes for patients with LEP requires our health-care systems to reengage at the provider level to implement interventions that ensure effective communication with patients with LEP and their families. Cheng and colleagues (2021) found many differences in family-centered rounds (FCR) with pediatric LEP families. They argue that FCRs for LEP families should be standardized, provide training for the team around LEP, increase access to interpreters, and redefine the roles of interpreters.[16] In addressing communication challenges, many studies emphasize the role of professional interpreters. Clinicians suggested improving comprehensive education and training programs for patients, families, and health-care professionals, along with integrating interpreters into ICU teams.[17] Sharma and colleagues (2023) showed the effectiveness of bicultural-bilingual caseworker patient navigators for patients with LEP.[18] These navigators bridge communication gaps and enhance knowledge, thus fostering equitable care. Thus, the role of a professional interpreter extends beyond verbatim translation; they should also become advocates, sensitively addressing cultural nuances to enhance the quality of care and overall experience for patients with LEP and their families.[15–18]

OUTCOMES

There are limited studies on clinical outcomes for patients with LEP relative to English-speaking patients. Although patients with LEP had no increased readmission risk after surgery/procedures, acute medical conditions,[19] or emergency department visits,[20] they were more likely to be readmitted after inpatient hospital stays for chronic medical conditions relative to their English-speaking counterparts.[19] Additionally, most studies have found no association between LEP and all-cause mortality.[19]

When patients with LEP are not effectively informed of their diagnosis and discharge instructions, they cannot fully participate in their care. This places them at a disadvantage and prevents them from reaching their optimal level of health. Squires and colleagues (2022) completed a retrospective cross-sectional study investigating the association of hospital readmission rates and language preferences of home care patients.[20] Continuity of care with the same nurse who did not speak the language of the patient with LEP showed a lower risk of readmission. When a team of health-care clinicians cannot provide effective communication, keeping consistent nurses with this patient population might prove beneficial.

There are similarly limited findings on adverse events for patients with LEP. There is no evidence that patients with LEP are more likely to experience adverse events.[19] However, a single-center study on inpatient safety events found that patients with LEP had a lower reported risk of patient safety events.[21] When diving deeper into these findings, the researchers find that this lower rate is due to fewer voluntary incident reports filed for patients with LEP. Importantly, they find no statistically significant difference in automatically reported incidents, suggesting that voluntary incident reporting may undercount safety events for patients with LEP.

There are mixed findings on the association between length of stay (LOS) and LEP. In a review of 17 studies on the topic, Woods and colleagues (2022) report that 9 studies (52.9%) found no difference in LOS, 4 studies (23.5%) found longer LOS for patients with LEP, 3 studies (17.6%) found shorter LOS for patients with LEP, and 1 study (5.9%) had mixed results. The authors suggest that these mixed findings on LOS may be mediated at the hospital level, and thus, single-center studies may have different findings.[19]

HEALTH-CARE COSTS

A few studies have compared hospital resource utilization and LOS between LEP and English-proficient patients. In a study of 80,404 critically ill patients from 2008 to 2017, who were discharged alive, patients with LEP had higher total costs for both ICU stay and overall hospital stay. Furthermore, non-US resident patients with LEP had higher overall costs compared with patients with LEP living in the United States, alluding to some possible cultural differences.[22]

A different study at a large academic medical center in Boston compared resource use between patients with LEP and English-speaking patients. It found that patients with LEP had an increased odd of being admitted after an emergency department (ED) encounter. Patients with LEP were also more likely to have x-rays and ultrasound orders than English-speaking patients. At the same time, the study identified that Spanish-speaking patients were less likely to be admitted than English-speaking patients. Among patients presenting with cardiovascular-related chief complaints, patients with LEP were more likely to have orders for stress tests compared with English-speaking patients.[20,23]

DISCUSSION AND FUTURE WORK

Reviewing the current state of the literature on this topic was difficult due to significant variations in the terminology used to describe this area of research.[24] We identified Medical Subject Heading and key search terms with a Knowledge Service expert. Our search terms to capture literature on this subject included the following:

1. Terms about language (languages, LEP, linguistically diverse, language proficiency, non-English speaking, and language barrier);
2. Terms about communication (communication, communication barrier, and suboptimal communication) and terms about disparities (health-care disparities, health-care inequities, equitable health-care, bias, inequity, and disparities); and
3. Terms about delivering health care to diverse populations (culturally competent care, professional family relations, and health-care delivery).

These search terms were broad and did not always overlap with each other. Without a standardized terminology for patients with LEP, it is more difficult to assess and add to the existing literature.

Much of the qualitative studies we reviewed highlighted the important role of an interpreter to not only be there for verbatim translation but also as an advocate to include cultural nuances, especially during important health-care decision-making. The studies on communication barriers mostly focused on end-of-life care in which the openness of the physician toward families with LEP, even with the presence of an interpreter, proved crucial.[10,11] In one study, physicians spent twice as much time with English-proficient families compared with patients with LEP, even with an interpreter.[14] Does cultural relevance and relatability cause this discrepancy? Do providers need cultural awareness training during such crucial decision-making that not only has physical impact on the patient but also has a mental and social impact on them and their families?[25]

However, these communication barriers exist long before conversations around end-of-life. Effective communication and health-care decision-making is necessary even before the patient is admitted into the hospital, as well as throughout their stay. A cohort study found that patients with LEP were more likely to be admitted to the hospital from an ED visit compared with English-speaking patients.[23] Was it because patients with LEP were sicker at presentation to the ED or was it because of a communication barrier? Data on the use of interpreters during the ED encounter would allow future studies to examine the impact of interpreter use.

A significant limitation in quantitative studies on patients with LEP is lack of consistent data collection. For example, at registration, language may not be accurately captured. Moreover, even if it is captured, patients who can "get by" speaking English but prefer to communicate in their native language may appear in the data as English-speaking, even if they are patients with LEP. Even beyond data collection on patient language, there is a significant lack of data on interpreter use during encounters with patients with LEP. Even in institutions that do capture this information, it is often collected as a dichotomous indicator of whether or not an interpreter was used during a patient encounter.[15,22] During an ICU stay, a patient will interact with many health-care providers, and the degree of interpreter use throughout the patient encounter is often unmeasured: Are interpreters used in every interaction? Are they only used at admission and discharge? Are they used during routine care? Are they used when some bilingual English-speaking family members are present that act as nonprofessional interpreters? The current data collection at many institutions leaves these questions unanswerable and thus quantitatively near impossible to study retrospectively.

SUMMARY

Collectively, the existing body of research on patients with LEP reveals a need for more attention to disparities in this population. Existing studies show mixed results regarding outcomes such as LOS, readmission rates, and all-cause mortality among patients with LEP, with elevated costs associated with factors such as prolonged mechanical ventilation, restraint use, and diagnostic testing. Research on end-of-life decision-making indicates a communication disparity, as physicians spend twice the time communicating with English-speaking family members compared with non-English-speaking counterparts, even with interpreters present. Some studies advocate for comprehensive interventions, including educational programs, training for families, patients, and health-care providers, and integrating interpreters into ICU rounds to improve communication and overall care quality for patients with LEP.

These findings highlight the complex challenges patients with LEP face in the health-care system, and the crucial need for targeted interventions to enhance language access, improve cultural competence among health-care professionals, and ensure equitable health-care outcomes for all patients. This includes educational and cultural training and interventions but also back-end interventions, such as standardized indicators of LEP and interpreter use in electronic health records. The reliable collection of these indicators will allow researchers to measure outcomes in this understudied population accurately.

CLINICS CARE POINTS

- Some studies advocate for comprehensive interventions, including educational programs, training for families, patients, and health-care providers, and integrating interpreters into ICU rounds to improve communication and overall care quality for patients with LEP.

- The findings highlight the complex challenges patients with LEP face in the health-care system, and the crucial need for targeted interventions to enhance language access, improve cultural competence among health-care professionals, and ensure equitable health-care outcomes for all patients.

- A significant limitation in quantitative studies on patients with LEP is the lack of consistent data collection, including patient language, English proficiency, and interpreter use throughout patient encounters.

ACKNOWLEDGMENTS

The authors would like to thank Laurie Regan, MLS, Senior Knowledge Service Specialist for her assistance with the literature search.

DISCLOSURE

The authors have nothing to disclose.

REFERENCES

1. Braveman P. What are health disparities and health equity? We need to be clear. Publ Health Rep 2014;129(Suppl 2):5–8.
2. Chichirez CM, Purcărea VL. Interpersonal communication in healthcare. J Med Life 2018;11(2):119–22.
3. HHS Headquarters. Civil Rights: Limited English Proficiency (LEP). U.S. Department of Health and Human Services: Washington, D.C. Available at: Limited English Proficiency (LEP) | HHS.govAccessed on November 12, 2023.
4. Haldar, S., Pillai, D., & Artiga, S. Overview of Health Coverage and Care for Individuals with Limited English Proficiency (LEP). KFF, Published: Jul 07, 2023. https://www.kff.org/racial-equity-and-health-policy/issue-brief/overview-of-health-coverage-and-care-for-individuals-with-limited-english-proficiency/#footnote-592615-6 Accessed on: November 12, 2023.
5. Hartford EA, Anderson AP, Klein EJ, et al. The Use and impact of professional interpretation in a pediatric emergency department. Acad Pediatr 2019;19(8):956–62.
6. Diamond L, Izquierdo K, Canfield D, et al. A systematic review of the impact of patient-physician non-English language concordance on quality of care and outcomes. J Gen Intern Med 2019;34(8):1591–606.
7. Diamond LC, Wilson-Stronks A, Jacobs EA. Do hospitals measure up to the national culturally and linguistically appropriate services standards? Med Care 2010;48(12):1080–7.
8. Diamond LC, Schenker Y, Curry L, et al. Getting by: underuse of interpreters by resident physicians. J Gen Intern Med 2009;24(2):256–62.
9. Espinoza Suarez NR, Urtecho M, Nyquist CA, et al. Consequences of suboptimal communication for patients with limited English proficiency in the intensive care unit and suggestions for a way forward: a qualitative study of healthcare team perceptions. J Crit Care 2021 Feb;61:247–51.
10. Barwise AK, Nyquist CA, Espinoza Suarez NR, et al. End-of-Life decision-making for ICU patients with limited English proficiency: a qualitative study of healthcare team insights. Crit Care Med 2019 Oct;47(10):1380–7.
11. Barwise A, Balls-Berry J, Soleimani J, et al. Interventions for end of life decision making for patients with limited English proficiency. J Immigr Minority Health 2020 Aug;22(4):860–72.
12. Yang C, Prokop L, Barwise A. Strategies used by healthcare systems to communicate with hospitalized patients and families with limited English proficiency during the COVID-19 pandemic: a narrative review. J Immigr Minority Health 2023; 25(6):1393–401.
13. Barwise A, Jaramillo C, Novotny P, et al. Differences in code status and end-of-life decision making in patients with limited English proficiency in the intensive care unit. Mayo Clin Proc 2018;93(9):1271–81.

14. Thornton JD, Pham K, Engelberg RA, et al. Families with limited English proficiency receive less information and support in interpreted intensive care unit family conferences. Crit Care Med 2009;37(1):89–95.
15. Ju M. Addressing health inequities for limited English proficiency patients: interpreter use and beyond. Pediatrics 2021;147(2). e2020032383.
16. Cheng JH, Wang C, Jhaveri V, et al. Health care provider practices and perceptions during family-centered rounds with limited English-proficient families. Acad Pediatr 2021;21(7):1223–9.
17. Suarez NRE, Urtecho M, Jubran S, et al. The Roles of medical interpreters in intensive care unit communication: a qualitative study. Patient Educ Counsel 2021;104(5):1100–8.
18. Sharma RK, Cowan A, Gill H, et al. Understanding the role of caseworker-cultural mediators in addressing healthcare inequities for patients with limited-English proficiency: a qualitative study. J Gen Intern Med 2023;38(5):1190–9.
19. Woods AP, Alonso A, Duraiswamy S, et al. Limited English proficiency and clinical outcomes after hospital-based care in English-speaking countries: a systematic review. J Gen Intern Med 2022;37(8):050–2061.
20. Squires A, Ma C, Miner S, et al. Assessing the influence of patient language preference on 30 day hospital readmission risk from home health care: a retrospective analysis. Int J Nurs Stud 2022;125:104093.
21. Schulson LB, Novack V, Folcarelli PH, et al. Inpatient patient safety events in vulnerable populations: a retrospective cohort study. BMJ Qual Saf 2020.
22. Barwise AK, Moriarty JP, Rosedahl JK, et al. Comparative costs for critically ill patients with limited English proficiency versus English proficiency. PLoS One 2023; 18(4):e0279126.
23. Schulson L, Novack V, Smulowitz PB, et al. Emergency department care for patients with limited English proficiency: a retrospective cohort study. J Gen Intern Med 2018;33(12):2113–9.
24. Ortega P, Shin TM, Martínez GA. Rethinking the term "limited English proficiency" to improve language-appropriate healthcare for all. J Immigr Minority Health 2022;24(3):799–805.
25. Lambert E, Strickland K, Gibson J. Cultural considerations at end-of-life for people of culturally and linguistically diverse backgrounds: a critical interpretative synthesis. J Clin Nurs 2023. https://doi.org/10.1111/jocn.16710.

Delirium and Coronavirus Disease 2019

Looking Back, Moving Forward

Kelly M. Potter, PhD, RN, CNE[a,*], Brenda T. Pun, DNP, RN[b],
Kerri Maya, PhD(c), MSL, RN, NPD-BC[c],
Bethany Young, PhD(c), RN, AGCNS-BC, CCRN[d],
Stacey Williams, DNP, APRN, CPNP-AC[e], Marc Schiffman, MD[f],
Annmarie Hosie, PhD, RN[g,h,i], Leanne M. Boehm, PhD, RN, ACNS-BC[j,k]

KEYWORDS

- Delirium • COVID-19 • ABCDEF bundle • Family engagement

CORONAVIRUS DISEASE 2019: CLINICAL CASE

In an intensive care unit (ICU) at the local community hospital, the team is caring for a 48-year-old male, 'David', with a history of chronic obstructive pulmonary disorder who lives at home with his wife and 2 children, ages 16 and 17. David presented to the hospital via the emergency room with severe shortness of breath, worsening over the last day, and an initial oxygen saturation of 84%. Over the course of just a few hours, David transitioned from requiring oxygen via nasal cannula to being intubated on 80% Fio_2 and a positive end-expiratory pressure (PEEP) of 14 cm H_2O. The hospital is at capacity, with all ICU beds filled with patients with similar presentations. David was admitted to a makeshift ICU that was converted from a patient overflow space. It is an ''all hands-on deck' situation for staff, with attending physicians and trainees from noncritical care settings on board to help care for coronavirus

[a] Department of Critical Care Medicine, CRISMA Center, University of Pittsburgh, Pittsburgh, PA, USA; [b] Department of Medicine, Pulmonary and Critical Care, Critical Illness, Brain Dysfunction, and Survivorship Center, Vanderbilt University Medical Center, Nashville, TN, USA; [c] Sutter Health System, Sacramento, CA, USA; [d] Hospital of the University of Pennsylvania, Philadelphia, PA, USA; [e] Monroe Carrell Jr Children's Hospital at Vanderbilt, Nashville, TN, USA; [f] Weill Cornell Medicine, New York, NY, USA; [g] School of Nursing & Midwifery Sydney, University of Notre Dame Australia, Sydney, New South Wales, Australia; [h] Cunningham Centre for Palliative Care, St Vincent's Health Network Sydney, Sydney, New South Wales, Australia; [i] IMPACCT- Improving Palliative, Aged and Chronic Care Through Research and Translation, University of Technology Sydney, Sydney, New South Wales, Australia; [j] School of Nursing, Vanderbilt University, Nashville, TN, USA; [k] Critical Illness, Brain Dysfunction, and Survivorship (CIBS) Center, Vanderbilt University Medical Center, Nashville, TN, USA
* Corresponding author. 100 Keystone Building, 3520 Fifth Avenue, Pittsburgh, PA 15213.
E-mail address: kelly.potter@pitt.edu

Crit Care Nurs Clin N Am 36 (2024) 415–426
https://doi.org/10.1016/j.cnc.2023.12.003
0899-5885/24/Crown Copyright © 2023 Published by Elsevier Inc. All rights reserved.
ccnursing.theclinics.com

KEY POINTS

- Occurrence of delirium, an acute neurocognitive condition characterized by disturbed attention, awareness, and cognition and associated with poor long-term outcomes, increased significantly in intensive care units (ICUs) during the coronavirus disease 2019 (COVID-19) pandemic due to increased sedation, immobilization, restraint use, isolation, and visitor restrictions.

- Full delivery of the ABCDEF (A = assess, prevent, and manage pain; B = both spontaneous awakening trials and spontaneous breathing trials; C = choice of analgesia and sedation; D = assess, prevent, and manage delirium; E = early mobility and exercise; F = family engagement and empowerment) bundle in ICUs is associated with a 40% lower likelihood of delirium compared with patients who receive partial implementation of the ABCDEF bundle, but implementation of the bundle stalled during the COVID-19 pandemic.

- Recruiting ABCDEF bundle champions may not only improve patient outcomes but also provide meaning, a sense of accomplishment, and increased work engagement among ICU clinicians—all strategies that may combat professional burnout.

- Novel care strategies that leverage informatics, the interprofessional team, and care coordination may facilitate better adherence to evidence-based care and reduce delirium and subsequent adverse outcomes among critically ill patients.

- The family is a vital component of critical care, and active opportunities for families to engage with their loved ones should be provided by clinicians and will reduce delirium-related agitation and distress.

disease 2019 (COVID-19) patients in the hospital's ICU. As the day progresses, David's oxygen levels remain low, and the team decides to place David in the prone position to enhance lung recruitment and medically paralyze him with cisatracurium to prevent him from breathing over the ventilator. The pharmacy is concerned about an impending shortage of propofol, so David is placed in a deep coma using midazolam and fentanyl. While David's paralytics are turned off a couple of days later, he remains sedated and restrained in bed, with his intravenous pump and monitors set outside the room to reduce the need for entry by staff, who provide direct care when fully covered in personal protective equipment. The hospital has a strict no-visitors policy to prevent transmission of the novel coronavirus. Seven days later, David's sedatives are titrated off and he self-extubates, thrashing in bed and unable to follow instructions. He is given haloperidol intravenously. Eight hours later he lies immobile in bed, unable to answer questions but maintaining eye contact.

DELIRIUM: A COMMON AND COMPLEX CLINICAL SYNDROME

The aforementioned clinical case describes a perfect recipe for the development of delirium during critical care. Delirium is an acute neurocognitive condition characterized by disturbed attention, awareness, and cognition. Predisposing factors (eg, comorbidities and cognitive impairment) and precipitating factors (eg, systemic illness and organ dysfunction, mechanical ventilation, benzodiazepines, opioids, immobilization, physical restraints) combine to increase the risk of delirium,[1] which then contributes to greater mortality, functional disability, and long-term cognitive impairment.[2,3] Throughout the COVID-19 pandemic, many patients, families, clinicians, and researchers in ICUs experienced severe distress due to the related devastation, which included increased rates of delirium. In this review, the authors describe the burden of delirium during the pandemic, the reversal of progress that had been made in delirium practices before the pandemic, and the journey we face to reduce this acute cognitive injury to critically ill patients moving forward.

HISTORICAL RECOGNITION OF DELIRIUM IN THE INTENSIVE CARE UNIT

In 1998, Dr Thomas L. Petty from the University of Colorado Health Sciences Center editorialized in *Chest* that, despite prior care where patients were awake and alert in the ICU, he now saw, "*paralyzed, sedated patients, lying without motion, appearing to be dead, except for the monitors that told [him] otherwise.*" The practice of using sedative medications to keep patients in unresponsive states where they "*appeared to be sleeping*" was common, arising from clinicians' benevolent desire that patients be comfortable on mechanical ventilation (or at least, forgetful of it), resulting in increased use of sedative-hypnotic agents in ICUs worldwide. Dr Petty described the resultant complications of deep sedation, including a "*clouded sensorium that often results in what has been termed as intensive care delirium.*" Researchers then began to recognize this as an acute iatrogenic brain injury, now commonly known as delirium. The early 2000s yielded valid and easy-to-use ICU delirium assessment tools for adults (eg, Confusion Assessment Method for the ICU [CAM-ICU], Intensive Care Delirium Screening Checklist).[4,5] A decade later pediatric ICU delirium screening tools were validated and published (eg, Pediatric CAM-ICU, Cornell Assessment of Pediatric Delirium).[6,7] The development of validated screening tools rapidly led to better understanding of ICU delirium prevalence, associated outcomes, and the development and testing of prevention and management interventions for both adults and children.[8,9]

ADVENT OF THE ABCDEF BUNDLE

In 2010, the ABCDEF bundle (A = assess, prevent, and manage pain; B = both spontaneous awakening trials and spontaneous breathing trials; C = choice of analgesia and sedation; D = assess, prevent, and manage delirium; E = early mobility and exercise; F = family engagement and empowerment) was proposed as a framework for ICU guideline implementation, integrating delirium assessment and management as part of this bundle of ICU evidence–based practices.[10,11] The ABCDEF bundle was foundational in understanding the interdependency of delirium prevention and management on sedation and mobility practices in addition to considering long-term recovery beginning in the ICU. The ABCDEF bundle, applicable to all patients in the ICU regardless of their admitting diagnosis or ventilation status, has been proven to be safe, efficacious, and feasible, with more complete performance yielding greater reductions in delirium, ventilator, and ICU days.[12] For example, in a study of over 15,000 critically ill adults, patients had a 40% lower likelihood of developing delirium when they received all components of the ABCDEF bundle compared with patients who received a lower proportion of bundled care.[12] The bundle was later adapted to meet the need for age-appropriate bundled delirium care for critically ill children.[13,14]

CORONAVIRUS DISEASE 2019S DISRUPTION OF ABCDEF BUNDLE IMPLEMENTATION

Due to strained staff, unprecedented patient volume, and limited resources, the COVID-19 pandemic disrupted progress made with ABCDEF bundle implementation. Not only did ABCDEF bundle adherence drop dramatically,[15] but practices also trended toward increased rates of delirium. Prolonged and deep sedation was commonly employed during the pandemic to manage agitation and ventilator-patient dyssynchrony while facilitating tolerance of higher PEEP and prone positioning. These practices aligned with early advocacy for neuromuscular blockade, which is inseparable from deep sedation, in the management of COVID-19 acute respiratory distress syndrome.[16] Consequently, patients with COVID-19 were prescribed higher doses of sedatives and analgesics than those without COVID-19. The percentage of physicians who regularly prescribed sedation increased from 86% to 94% and the percentage who performed daily awakening trials decreased from up to 66% to 30%.[17,18] Reports of propofol shortages, prolonged neuromuscular blockade, prone ventilation, and concerns about propofol infusion syndrome also increased the reliance on benzodiazepines, a known deliriogenic drug, leading to patients with COVID-19 receiving benzodiazepines for a median of 7 (4–12) days.[16]

Along with increased sedative administration, patients had less physical and social contact with health care providers, were more often restrained in bed, were less mobile and unable to leave their rooms, and were cared for by stressed staff who were hard to recognize due to personal protective equipment (**Fig. 1**). Clinicians may have also been advised by hospital leadership to limit patient interactions to conserve personal protective equipment.[19] These factors, combined with limited or nonexistent hospital visitation, meant patients had fewer family members physically present with them, which likely contributed to the increased use of physical restraints.[20] Persistently elevated restraint use, which acutely increased at the beginning of the pandemic, was reported even months after the initial wave.[21] Additionally, the pandemic intensified barriers to early mobilization, a practice that has positive and synergistic effects on ICU patient outcomes when paired with other ABCDEF bundle components. In an analysis of global ICU practices, COVID-19 infection was not itself a major barrier to mobilization; rather, mechanical ventilation and other associated clinical therapies (eg, deep sedation) decreased the likelihood of mobilization.[22]

Thus, rates of delirium increased, affecting up to 84% of adult COVID-19 patients[23–25] compared to up to 30% of critically ill patients pre-pandemic.[26] Those

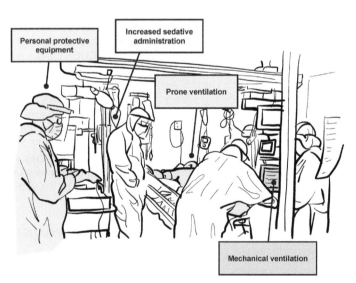

Fig. 1. Crisis changes in clinical care during the coronavirus disease 2019 pandemic, including the increased use of personal protective equipment, deep sedation, prone ventilation, and mechanical ventilation, contributed to double the occurrence of delirium in the intensive care unit.

diagnosed with COVID-19 had 4.42 (95% confidence interval [CI] 2.69–7.26) greater odds of developing delirium as compared to non–COVID-19 patients, although delirium incidence did not differ among those with 2 or more days of mechanical ventilation.[24] Likewise, COVID-19 patients with delirium also experienced worse outcomes than their non-delirious counterparts, with 3.2 (95% CI 2.1–4.8) greater odds of short-term mortality in those with delirium compared to those without.[27]

Similar trends occurred in the pediatric setting. The gains in evidence-based pediatric critical care using the ABCDEF bundle (64% pre-pandemic) were not sustained.[28] While the literature describing the influence of COVID-19 on pediatric ICU delirium care is scarce, reports indicate the rate of moderate to severe COVID-19 was dramatically less than in adults.[29] Rather, children who had multiple comorbidities were more likely to have moderate to severe COVID-19 or multisystem inflammatory syndrome in children that resulted in ICU care, although these cases represented less than 30% of all pediatric ICU cases.[30] Still, pediatric patients experienced similar increase in immobilization, isolation, analgosedation, and visitor restrictions, contributing to worse disorientation and late recognition of delirium.[31–33]

WHERE ARE WE NOW?

Now, nearly 4 years after the pandemic began, the health care system faces different challenges. While present COVID-19 surges are nothing compared to the high numbers in 2020, we still find ourselves navigating such surges and recovering from collateral damage from the height of the quarantine isolation and chaos of high volumes. Specifically, in many of our ICUs, we face significant staffing shortages leading to strained systems, high workload, and burnout. The strain on staff contributes to poor implementation and disconnect with evidence-based practice, including the ABCDEF bundle. Many ICUs continue practices started during the pandemic, originally intended to be exclusive to COVID-19 patients, with all patients, such as deep sedation, prone ventilation, and limited visitation hours. All these practices sustain the burden of delirium and coma during critical illness.

HOW DO WE MOVE FORWARD?

Going forward, we make the same call as Dr Petty in his editorial 25 years ago: "We must return to the basic principles of human caring and the fundamental principle of reason, as we try to guide desperately ill patients along the pathway to recovery." While we have equipment and medication that can support critically ill patients in times of need, "supportive care" can also result in devastating cognitive impairment that persists for years after the acute illness. No pharmacologic or mechanical advance "can begin to replace the caring physician, nurse, and therapist at the bedside to bring a patient from the threshold of death, back to the living." Therefore, we call for the resuscitation of ABCDEF-bundled care for adults and children by empowering clinical champions to promote uptake, implementing creative and novel care strategies to foster a team environment that promotes holistic recovery, and reintegrating patient-centered approaches in our new era of critical care (**Fig. 2**).

Motivating Champions of Care

We must address the ongoing moral distress experienced by many health care workers to create a care environment, where teams are motivated to pursue high-quality care. Persistent burnout, compassion fatigue, and low levels of personal accomplishment linger from the pandemic and negatively impact nurse professional commitment, clinical performance, and attitudes.[34,35] However, renewed vigilance around the ABCDEF

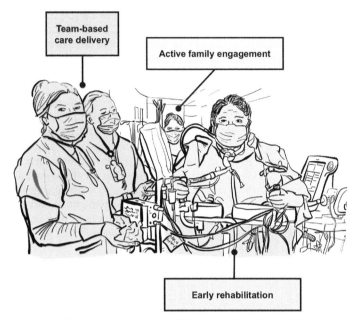

Fig. 2. Resuscitation of patient-centered care after coronavirus disease 2019 should emphasize motivating champions of the ABCDEF bundle, including the family as an active partner in care, and integrating novel care models that emphasize the strengths of the interprofessional team. (A = assess, prevent, and manage pain; B = both spontaneous awakening trials and spontaneous breathing trials; C = choice of analgesia and sedation; D = assess, prevent, and manage delirium; E = early mobility and exercise; F = family engagement and empowerment).

bundle could be a strategy to combat professional burnout. Mastery experiences, which include learning new things, are associated with higher work engagement for ICU nurses.[36] Transforming nurses into delirium prevention experts could be a strategy to provide meaning, a sense of accomplishment, and increased work engagement. Creating experts begins with standardized education about ABCDEF bundle protocols. Standardized education equips nurses and other health care team members to advocate for high-quality, evidence-based patient care.[37] Attention to the ABCDEF bundle may also transform exhaustion with the unwieldy problem of the pandemic into renewed energy directed at providing holistic care to individual human beings. The ABCDEF bundle provides tangible interventions to prevent delirium, a stark contrast to the distress of being underequipped to proactively meet patient needs during the pandemic.[38]

Novel Care Strategies

We must amplify what we have learned in past efforts to facilitate care coordination and implementation of evidence-based delirium care, while also recognizing that the critical care environment is different from its pre-pandemic state. Fatigue is common among ICU clinicians, and worse when compounded by burnout. Clinical decision support tools, like checklists and automated prompting, may help facilitate adherence to evidence-based delirium care.[39,40] Informatics and data science can be leveraged to reduce alert fatigue by providing customized feedback, prompts, or recommendations tailored to the clinician, patient, and setting. Thus, these systems may not add to the psychological burden faced by clinicians.[41] The design of such systems should emphasize how clinicians interact with the computer, electronic health literacy, and education priorities to facilitate their use.[42,43]

Pre-pandemic, organizational factors were the most commonly reported barriers to ABCDEF bundle implementation, including team structure.[44–46] When more members of the interdisciplinary team are involved in the individual components of the ABCDEF bundle, it is more likely that these components are implemented routinely, yet rarely does this occur.[47] Inclusion of the entire interprofessional team, including the family, social workers, pharmacists, psychologists, palliative care specialists, chaplains, and respiratory and rehabilitation therapists (physical, occupational, and speech), may help clinicians generate an optimal plan of care that promotes ABCDEF bundle implementation. However, given the turnover and structural changes among the ICU team since the pandemic, a robust analysis of how organizational factors and team dynamics influence individual contributions to ABCDEF implementation by health care team members is urgently needed to inform implementation strategy selection geared toward sustainability.

Both adult and pediatric patients who develop delirium are at high risk for post-intensive care syndrome (PICS)[48–50] and should receive early referral to post-ICU recovery programs.[51–53] ICU recovery care coordination via a multidisciplinary outpatient clinic, staffed by health care team members specializing in PICS, provides individualized evaluation, management, and referral to address ongoing needs often missed in standard ICU follow-up.[54] Akin to a navigator program, ICU recovery clinics assist patients and family members with long-term recovery and provide support and guidance to those affected by delirium, aiding in adaptation to post-ICU life. More importantly, ICU staff involvement in ICU recovery programs offers benefits across the critical illness continuum by providing targets for ICU-based quality improvement initiatives, creating roles for ICU survivors to volunteer within the ICU setting, sensitizing ICU team members to the realities of PICS and the patient/family experience, and improving the meaningfulness of ICU work by creating a feedback loop.[55]

Reimagining Family Engagement

Finally, we must reimagine opportunities for enhanced family inclusion in our ICUs—with an emphasis on the *art*, not just the science, of critical care.[56] While COVID-19 highlighted deficiencies in hospital communication, in reality, these limitations have always existed. Nevertheless, family engagement and empowerment are integral components of the ABCDEF bundle of ICU care.

Families of critically ill patients may face barriers to in-person presence because of geographic distance, work or caregiving responsibilities, economic hardship, transportation challenges, or health limitations.[57] Given pre-existing constraints on visitation, even without considering hospital restrictions, we must use best practices to communicate and facilitate family engagement and empowerment at a distance. While both the health care team and family members generally favor in-person conversations, empathy can successfully be conveyed via a phone or video. Advanced logistical planning can also facilitate family engagement with programs like VoiceLove, a virtual health care visitation system being researched and funded by the National Institute of Aging and the National Institute of Mental Health. Such technologies offer an opportunity to greatly enhance family connection while simultaneously relieving this time-consuming task from the nursing staff. Communication with family members at a distance can be further improved by assigning a point person to receive updates for continuity, frequently evaluating family understanding, allowing the family to view the patient and their surroundings via videos, and offering time for the patient to interact with their family without health care team members present.[57,58]

When in-person, family members want to actively participate in care and prefer talking, providing music, reading aloud, hygiene-related or medical-related activities, completing bed changes, bathing, or suctioning the patient over passive activities like receiving information.[59] While there is limited evidence on the benefits of familiar voices for managing delirium, some investigators have concluded that auditory stimulation, particularly, direct auditory stimulation through talking to the patient, might be useful for improving the recovery of consciousness and increasing the arousal of comatose patients.[60] In addition, others have indicated that family member voices can increase level of consciousness of comatose patients with traumatic brain injury and acute subdural hematoma.[61] However, like how burnout and poor staffing impact the implementation of the overall ABCDEF bundle, high staff-to-patient ratios and burnout influence how health care team members facilitate opportunities to activate family members. Managing barriers often must begin at the organizational level, but a facilitated understanding of the value of family presence (eg, reduced delirium-related agitation and distress) may increase team member willingness to offer opportunities for family members to participate in care.[62,63]

Coordinated, early care pathways for family support also improve communication and patient-centeredness and family-centeredness, which are markers of improved decision-making that may contribute to value-concordant care. ICUs should develop policies and standards of care for identifying and addressing patient and family distress. Family members should be empowered with comprehensive education about delirium, emphasizing its presentation and potentially distressing symptoms, the family's role in its management (eg, assisting with orientation activities and mobility), and its significance in the care process. The "VALUE" mnemonic (Value family statements, Acknowledge emotions, Listen, Understand the patient as a person, and Elicit questions) can be implemented to enhance communication, foster empathy, and establish a collaborative atmosphere between the health care team and family.[64] These strategies ensure the well-being of both patients and families is adequately considered and addressed, contributing to a holistic patient-centered and family-centered approach to ICU delirium care.

MOVING FORWARD

Patients, families, and clinicians collectively confronted often overwhelming challenges because of the COVID-19 pandemic. Crisis changes in clinical practice resulted in increased sedation, isolation, restraint use, visitor restrictions, and de-adoption of the ABCDEF bundle, resulting in rates of delirium double those seen pre-pandemic. Clinicians, now burnt out and distressed, face the vital task of moving forward after the pandemic. Clinicians must be supported by their leadership and ICU environments to reenergize and champion the ABCDEF bundle, deliver critical care using models that facilitate recovery after critical illness without additional burden, and emphasize the art of clinical care. The path forward requires us to both look back to where we came from and move ahead with common goals in mind, including to reduce the burden of delirium and cognitive impairment among patients and to promote the well-being of their families.

FUNDING

K.M. Potter, was supported by the NIH (T32HL007820) during the preparation of this manuscript.

CLINICS CARE POINTS

- As a result of the COVID-19 pandemic, occurrence of delirium in the ICU has increased compared to pre-pandemic.
- Routine use of deep sedation, immobilization, restraint use, and isolation and visitor restriction contribute to the burden of delirium and risks of mortality and long-term functional and cognitive impairment.
- The resuscitation of patient-centered care requires ABCDEF bundle champions to promote uptake, novel care strategies that foster evidence-based and interprofessional care, and humane approaches that actively integrate the family as a necessary component of critical care.

REFERENCES

1. Ormseth C, LaHue S, Oldham M, et al. Predisposing and precipitating factors associated with delirium: a systematic review. JAMA Netw Open 2023;6(1):e2249950.
2. Ely E, Shintani A, Truman B, et al. Delirium as a predictor of mortality in mechanically ventilated patients in the intensive care unit. JAMA 2004;291(14):1753–62.
3. Pandharipande P, Girard T, Jackson J, et al. Long-term cognitive impairment after critical illness. N Engl J Med 2013;369(14):1306–16.
4. Ely E, Inouye S, Bernard G, et al. Delirium in mechanically ventilated patients: validity and reliability of the confusion assessment method for the intensive care unit (CAM-ICU). JAMA 2001;286(21):2703–10.
5. Bergeron N, Dubois M, Dumont M, et al. Intensive care delirium screening checklist: evaluation of a new screening tool. Intensive Care Med 2001;27(5):859–64.
6. Smith H, Boyd J, Fuchs D, et al. Diagnosing delirium in critically ill children: validity and reliability of the pediatric confusion assessment method for the intensive care unit. Crit Care Med 2011;39(1):150–7.
7. Traube C, Silver G, Kearney J, et al. Cornell Assessment of Pediatric Delirium: a valid, rapid, observational tool for screening delirium in the PICU. Crit Care Med 2014;42(3):656–63.
8. Kalvas L, Harrison T. State of the science in pediatric ICU delirium: an integrative review. Res Nurs Health 2020;43(4):341–55.
9. van den Boogaard M, Slooter A. Delirium in critically ill patients: current knowledge and future perspectives. BJA Educ 2019;19(12):398–404.
10. Devlin JW, Skrobik Y, Gelinas C, et al. Clinical practice guidelines for the prevention and management of pain, agitation/sedation, delirium, immobility, and sleep disruption in adult patients in the ICU. Crit Care Med 2018;46(9):e825–73.
11. Vasilevskis EE, Ely EW, Speroff T, et al. Reducing iatrogenic risks: ICU-acquired delirium and weakness–crossing the quality chasm. Chest 2010;138(5):1224–33.
12. Pun B, Balas M, Barnes-Daly M, et al. Caring for critically ill patients with the ABCDEF bundle: results of the ICU liberation collaborative in over 15,000 adults. Crit Care Med 2019;47(1):3–14.
13. Engel J, von BF, Baumgartner I, et al. Modified ABCDEF-bundles for critically ill pediatric patients - what could they look like? Front Pediatr 2022;10:886334.
14. Smith H, Besunder J, Betters K, et al. Society of critical care medicine clinical practice guidelines on prevention and management of pain, agitation, neuromuscular blockade, and delirium in critically ill pediatric patients with consideration of

the ICU environment and early mobility. Pediatr Crit Care Med 2022;23(2): e74–110.

15. Liu K, Nakamura K, Katsukawa H, et al. Implementation of the ABCDEF bundle for critically ill ICU patients during the COVID-19 pandemic: a multi-National 1-day point prevalence study. Front Med 2021;8:735860.

16. Pun B, Badenes R, Heras L, et al. Prevalence and risk factors for delirium in critically ill patients with COVID-19 (COVID-D): a multicentre cohort study. Lancet Respir Med 2021;9(3):239–50.

17. Morandi A, Piva S, Ely E, et al. Worldwide survey of the "assessing pain, both spontaneous awakening and breathing trials, choice of drugs, delirium monitoring/management, early exercise/mobility, and family empowerment" (ABCDEF) bundle. Crit Care Med 2017;45(11).

18. Luz M, Brandão BB, de C, et al, REV. Practices in sedation, analgesia, mobilization, delirium, and sleep deprivation in adult intensive care units (SAMDS-ICU): an international survey before and during the COVID-19 pandemic. Ann Intensive Care 2022;12(1):9.

19. Rosen A, Carter D, Applebaum J, et al. Critical care clinicians' experiences of patient safety during the COVID-19 pandemic. J Patient Saf 2022;18(8):e1219–25.

20. Font R, Quintana S, Monistrol O. Impact of family restrictions during COVID-19 pandemic on the use of physical restraint in an acute hospital: an observational study. J Healthc Qual Res 2021;36(5):263–8.

21. Jones A, Goodarzi Z, Lee J, et al. Chemical and physical restraint use during acute care hospitalization of older adults: a retrospective cohort study and time series analysis. PLoS One 2022;17(10):e0276504.

22. Liu K, Nakamura K, Kudchadkar S, et al. Mobilization and rehabilitation practice in ICUs during the COVID-19 pandemic. J Intensive Care Med 2022;37(9): 1256–64.

23. Helms J, Kremer S, Merdji H, et al. Delirium and encephalopathy in severe COVID-19: a cohort analysis of ICU patients. Crit Care 2020;24(1). s13054-020-03200-1.

24. Westphal G, Fernandes R, Pereira A, et al. Incidence of delirium in critically ill patients with and without COVID-19. J Intensive Care Med 2023;38(8):751–9.

25. Bernard-Valnet R, Favre E, Bernini A, et al. Delirium in adults with COVID-19-related acute respiratory distress syndrome: comparison with other etiologies. Neurology 2022;99(20):e2326–35.

26. Krewulak K, Stelfox H, Leigh J, et al. Incidence and prevalence of delirium subtypes in an adult ICU: a systematic review and meta-analysis. Crit Care Med 2018;46(12):2029–35.

27. Shao S, Lai C, Chen Y, et al. Prevalence, incidence and mortality of delirium in patients with COVID-19: a systematic review and meta-analysis. Age Ageing 2021;50(5):1445–53.

28. Ista E, Redivo J, Kananur P, et al. ABCDEF bundle practices for critically ill children: an international survey of 161 PICUs in 18 countries. Crit Care Med 2022; 50(1):114–25.

29. Kim L, Whitaker M, O'Halloran A, et al. Hospitalization rates and characteristics of children aged< 18 years hospitalized with laboratory-confirmed COVID-19—COVID-NET, 14 states, March 1–July 25, 2020. MMWR (Morb Mortal Wkly Rep) 2020;69(32):1081.

30. Kompaniyets L, Agathis N, Nelson J, et al. Underlying medical conditions associated with severe COVID-19 illness among children. JAMA Netw Open 2021; 4(6):e2111182.

31. Castro R, Rodríguez-Rubio M, Magalhães-Barbosa M, et al. Pediatric delirium in times of COVID-19. Rev Bras Ter Intensiva 2022;33(4):483–6.

32. Sisk B, Cull W, Harris JM, et al. National trends of cases of COVID-19 in children based on US state health department data. Pediatrics 2020;146(6).

33. Pumphrey K, Bouzaher A, Achuff B-J, et al. Sedation practices in the PICU: an unexpected casualty of COVID-19. Critical Care Explorations 2022;4(6).

34. Alharbi J, Jackson D, Usher K. The potential for COVID-19 to contribute to compassion fatigue in critical care nurses. J Clin Nurs 2020;29(15–16):2762–4.

35. Galanis P, Vraka I, Fragkou D, et al. Nurses' burnout and associated risk factors during the COVID-19 pandemic: a systematic review and meta-analysis. J Adv Nurs 2021;77(8):3286–302.

36. Haruna Y, Shiromaru M, Sumikawa M. Factors related to intensive care unit Nurses' work engagement: a web-based survey. Nurs Health Sci 2023;25(3):445–55.

37. Albert B. Prevention as intervention: reducing incident delirium in heart failure. J Dr Nurs Pract 2019;12(2):159–88.

38. González-Gil M, González-Blázquez C, Parro-Moreno A, et al. Nurses' perceptions and demands regarding COVID-19 care delivery in critical care units and hospital emergency services. Intensive Crit Care Nurs 2021;62:102966.

39. King A, Potter K, Seaman J, et al. Measuring performance on the ABCDEF bundle during interprofessional rounds via a nurse-based assessment tool. Am J Crit Care 2023;32(2):92–9.

40. King A, Angus D, Cooper G, et al. A voice-based digital assistant for intelligent prompting of evidence-based practices during ICU rounds. J Biomed Inform 2023;146:104483.

41. King A, Kahn J. The role of data science in closing the implementation gap. Crit Care Clin 2023;39(4):701–16.

42. Gray K, Slavotinek J, Dimaguila G, et al. Artificial intelligence education for the health workforce: expert survey of approaches and needs. JMIR Med Educ 2022;8(2):e35223.

43. Malerbi F, Nakayama L, Gayle D R, et al. Digital education for the deployment of artificial intelligence in health care. J Med Internet Res 2023;25:e43333.

44. Boehm L, Pun B, Stollings J, et al. A multisite study of nurse-reported perceptions and practice of ABCDEF bundle components. Intensive Crit Care Nurs 2020;60:102872.

45. Costa DK, White MR, Ginier E, et al. Identifying barriers to delivering the awakening and breathing coordination, delirium, and early exercise/mobility bundle to minimize adverse outcomes for mechanically ventilated patients: a systematic review. Chest 2017;152(2):304–11.

46. Boltey E, Iwashyna T, Hyzy R, et al. Ability to predict team members' behaviors in ICU teams is associated with routine ABCDE implementation. J Crit Care 2019;51:192–7.

47. Costa D, Valley T, Miller M, et al. ICU team composition and its association with ABCDE implementation in a quality collaborative. J Crit Care 2018;44:1–6.

48. Manning J, Pinto N, Rennick J, et al. Conceptualizing post intensive care syndrome in children-the PICS-p framework. Pediatr Crit Care Med 2018;19(4):298–300.

49. Watson R, Choong K, Colville G, et al. Life after critical illness in children-toward an understanding of pediatric post-intensive care syndrome. J Pediatr 2018;198:16–24.

50. Hiser S, Fatima A, Ali M, et al. Post-intensive care syndrome (PICS): recent updates. J Intensive Care 2023;11(1):23.

51. Sayde G, Stefanescu A, Hammer R. Interdisciplinary treatment for survivors of critical illness due to COVID-19: expanding the post-intensive care recovery model and impact on psychiatric outcomes. J Acad Consult Liaison Psychiatry 2023;64(3):226–35.
52. Mikkelsen M, Still M, Anderson B, et al. Society of critical care medicine's international consensus conference on prediction and identification of long-term impairments after critical illness. Crit Care Med 2020;48(11).
53.. Hall TA, Greene RK, Lee JB, et al. Post-intensive care syndrome in a cohort of school-aged children and adolescent ICU survivors: the importance of follow-up in the acute recovery phase. J Pediatr Intensive Care 2022;36(3):639–63.
54. Bloom S, Stollings J, Kirkpatrick O, et al. Randomized clinical trial of an ICU recovery pilot program for survivors of critical illness. Crit Care Med 2019;47(10): 1337–45.
55. Haines KJ, Sevin CM, Hibbert E, et al. Key mechanisms by which post-ICU activities can improve in-ICU care: results of the international THRIVE collaboratives. Intensive Care Med 2019;45(7):939–47.
56. MA H. The arts unique to critical care nursing: hard to measure but breathtakingly manifest in a pandemic. Dimens Crit Care Nurs 2020;39(5):287–9.
57. Milner K. Evolution of visiting the intensive care unit. Crit Care Clin 2023;39(3): 541–58.
58. Kennedy N, Steinberg A, Arnold R, et al. Perspectives on telephone and video communication in the intensive care unit during COVID-19. Annals of the American Thoracic Society 2021;18(5):838–47.
59. Hetland B, McAndrew N, Kupzyk K, et al. Family caregiver preferences and contributions related to patient care in the ICU. West J Nurs Res 2022;44(3):214–26.
60. Park S, Davis A. Effectiveness of direct and non-direct auditory stimulation on coma arousal after traumatic brain injury. Int J Nurs Pract 2016;22(4):391–6.
61. Tavangar H, Shahriary-Kalantary M, Salimi T, et al. Effect of family members' voice on level of consciousness of comatose patients admitted to the intensive care unit: a single-blind randomized controlled trial. Adv Biomed Res 2015;4:106.
62. Eggenberger S, Sanders M. A family nursing educational intervention supports nurses and families in an adult intensive care unit. Aust Crit Care 2016;29(4): 217–23.
63. Lee Y, Lee J, Kim J, et al. Non-pharmacological nursing interventions for prevention and treatment of delirium in hospitalized adult patients: systematic review of randomized controlled trials. Int J Environ Res Publ Health 2021;18(16):8853.
64. Davidson J, Aslakson R, Long A, et al. Guidelines for family-centered care in the neonatal, pediatric, and adult ICU. Crit Care Med 2017;45(1):103–28.

Connecting the Dots

Unveiling the Overlapping Realities of Long Coronavirus Disease and Post-Intensive Care Syndrome

Danielle Gott, MSN, RN[a],*, Katherine Orsillo, MSN, RN[a],
Amberly Ticotsky, MPH, BSN, RN[b]

KEYWORDS

- COVID-19 • Long COVID • Post-acute sequelae of COVID-19
- Post-intensive care syndrome • Survivorship • Survivorship prog

KEY POINTS

- The coronavirus disease 2019 (COVID-19) pandemic brought unprecedented numbers of patients to our intensive care units, many of whom continue(d) to have sequelae well beyond their admission.
- Sequelae often take the form of post-acute sequelae of COVID-19 (PASC) and/or post-intensive care syndrome (PICS); both are difficult to define syndromes that are often overlooked by providers.
- Multidisciplinary, coordinated care is necessary for the optimal treatment of both PASC and PICS.
- Further research and attention are needed for both PASC and PICS.

INTRODUCTION

In the early days of the coronavirus disease 2019 (COVID-19) pandemic, intensive care units (ICUs) across the globe were stretched to their limits with an influx of critically ill patients, many requiring prolonged periods of invasive ventilation, sedation, and other life-sustaining treatments. In Massachusetts, over 1000 patients with COVID-19 required ICU level of care by April 2020, necessitating many hospitals to expand their critical care areas to accommodate this surge of patients.[1] At Beth Israel Deaconess Medical Center (BIDMC), a 743-bed academic medical center in Boston, ICU capacity increased by 93%, from 77 beds to 149 beds at its peak during this time.[2]

[a] Professional Development, Beth Israel Deaconess Medical Center, 330 Brookline Avenue, Rabb 244C, Boston, MA 02215, USA; [b] Critical Illness and COVID-19 Survivorship Program, Beth Israel Deaconess Medical Center, 330 Brookline Avenue, Boston, MA 02215, USA
* Corresponding author. 330 Brookline Avenue, Boston, MA 02115.
E-mail address: dcgott@bidmc.harvard.edu

Crit Care Nurs Clin N Am 36 (2024) 427–436
https://doi.org/10.1016/j.cnc.2023.12.006
0899-5885/24/© 2023 Elsevier Inc. All rights reserved.

ccnursing.theclinics.com

Although a complex issue, a major stressor to ICU capacity at BIDMC was the lengthy ICU stay of critically ill patients with COVID-19. Even when these patients had improved sufficiently to transition to an alternate level of care, they continued to face a long road ahead in their recovery. Over time, it became clear that these patients would require continued support, and thus the medical center's Critical Illness and COVID-19 Survivorship Program (Survivorship Program) was created with the aim of providing this ongoing care.

Initially, the program was focused on the risk of post-intensive care syndrome (PICS), a group of impairments in physical function, cognition, and mental health that may persist long after an ICU admission. Over time, however, a new concern also emerged with the identification of post-acute sequelae of COVID-19 (PASC), or what is colloquially referred to as long COVID. Patients outside of intensive care, even those who did not require hospitalization, were noted to also be experiencing lingering symptoms, some very similar to those experienced as a consequence of PICS. Therefore, the Survivorship Program expanded to also serve this patient population with a multidisciplinary, coordinated approach to care. This article will aim to share key points and lessons learned over the past 3 years in the Survivorship Program, highlight 3 common symptoms of PASC and PICS, as well as look toward to the future of care for patients after COVID-19 infection and/or critical illness.

BACKGROUND
Postintensive Care Syndrome

Throughout surges of the COVID-19 pandemic, acute care settings were stretched beyond their limits when caring for the critically ill COVID-19 patient population. Unprecedented numbers of critically ill patients were hospitalized in an ICU setting throughout the world. Fortunately, due to groundbreaking advances in science and effective treatments for COVID-19 patients, there was a dramatic increase in the number of patients who survived critical illness.[3] However, these survivors were at an increased risk of developing long-standing sequelae and PICS.

Patients who survive an ICU admission and are later discharged often have many long-standing impairments. Although PICS is not unique to a COVID-19 diagnosis, it has certainly become one of the foremost triggers of intensive care admissions over the past several years and has thus shed light on this often invisible illness. The Society of Critical Care Medicine, in 2010, coined the term PICS to describe the impairments that occur after a critical illness and an ICU admission.[4] PICS, while difficult to objectively diagnose, is defined as "new onset or worsening of impairment(s) in physical, cognitive, and/or mental health that arose after the ICU and persisted beyond hospital discharge."[5]

Survivors of critical care admissions are also at an increased risk for hospital readmission and diagnoses of an acute or worsened chronic illness. In addition, these patients have a higher risk of death in the years following a critical care stay.[6] More than half of all those who experience an ICU admission will go on to develop the constellation of symptoms known as PICS. Patients often experience long-term cognitive, physical, or mental health symptoms for several months to years following an ICU admission.[5,7] ICU survivors who develop PICS report a significant symptom burden, such as pain, fatigue, depression, anxiety, and post-traumatic stress, which affects their quality of life, ability to remain employed, and their potential to reclaim their independence.[6]

With each surge of COVID-19, frontline medical staff caring for patients admitted to the ICU grew increasingly concerned for the future debilitation that these patients would suffer after, and only if, their patients survived their ICU admission. Many studies have established the clinical outcomes for patients following ICU treatment for COVID-19 to be significant. One year after an ICU admission for COVID-19, those still experiencing physical symptoms have been reported at 74.3%, mental symptoms reported at 26.2%, and cognitive symptoms at 16.2%.[8] Another study showed that the prevalence of PICS after an ICU admission for COVID-19 to be higher than that of typical ICU admissions, with at least half of all post-ICU COVID-19 patients experiencing PICS at 6 months, while other studies have demonstrated that an estimated 90% to 91% of COVID-19 ICU patients experienced at least 1 aspect of PICS long after discharge.[3,9]

It is evident that PICS is common among COVID-19 ICU survivors. Although appropriate primary care follow-up after an ICU admission is achievable, post-ICU recovery programs, like the one established at BIDMC, were developed in response to long-term disabilities faced by patients experiencing PICS to better manage these patients' symptoms by a variety of interprofessional team members.[10] Eaton and colleagues[6] concluded that post-ICU recovery programs should focus on symptom management, social and spiritual support, and care planning to assist in assessing and treating PICS. It is necessary to improve care for these patients after they have experienced the severe, acute phase of illness of COVID-19. Follow-up care and care planning through a survivorship program for this patient population can have positive effects for patients and their symptoms of PICS following a COVID-19 ICU admission.

Long Coronavirus Disease

In January 2020, reports began to circulate that a new rapidly spreading novel coronavirus (COVID-19) had been identified. This virus predominately caused acute respiratory distress and created a worldwide pandemic. Health care systems became overwhelmed, and millions of lives have been greatly impacted. While the acute phase of the COVID-19 virus has evolved and progressed to be more often an illness that is quite mild and mainly managed outside of the hospital, there are a growing number of people who are impacted well beyond their acute infection.[11] These lingering and new symptoms that persist after any severity of a COVID-19 infection have become a public health and financial concern.[12] Now known as PASC, or long COVID, more than 200 symptoms involving multiple organs have been identified as part of this post-viral illness.[13] These long-lasting symptoms are debilitating and can occur in the absence of preexisting conditions or medical explanation. Long COVID has garnered worldwide attention with substantial prevalence. In fact, at least 14% of US adults report having suffered lingering post–COVID-19 symptoms, although many estimate this number to be much higher.[14] Additionally, long COVID impacts a patient's ability to participate in the workforce with economic impacts.[15] For this reason, attention to this matter is necessary. Ongoing research at both the federal and international levels is warranted.

Like PICS, defining long COVID is difficult due to the large number of symptoms and the potential for overlapping diagnoses. While there has been an initial development of a definition, there remains no concrete diagnostic test, and long COVID remains poorly understood.[16,17] There is still work to be done before final diagnostic criteria can be identified. Research is currently underway related to many different aspects of long COVID. At this point, however, it has been established that long COVID can include an exacerbation of previous symptoms and/or a new constellation of concerns. These symptoms persist at least 4 weeks after an infection and often involve symptoms such as physical and mental fatigue, cognitive deficits, as well as mental health concerns.

DISCUSSION

As there is no current definition of long COVID and no definitive testing to be done, long COVID programs have charted their own course. PICS, in a similar way, has some guideposts, but no clear program to recovery. Because of this, it can be challenging for patients with long COVID or PICS to find providers that legitimize and affirm their symptoms. Often diagnosed with anxiety or another mental health issue, their concerns for fatigue or brain fog can be overlooked. Therefore, validating patients is a core component of the Survivorship Program at BIDMC. Drawing on prior knowledge of similar diseases like chronic fatigue syndrome, other post-viral illnesses, dysautonomia, and postural orthostatic tachycardia syndrome, as well as specialty expertise, the Survivorship Program at BIDMC uses a collaborative referral process with a rehabilitation focus to evaluate and provide support for patients' symptoms. Leveraging specialists across the health care network and having regular case discussions and provider collaboration has allowed the work to alleviate symptoms, even when the disease process is not fully understood. This interdisciplinary team has found some success with treating patients' symptoms and supporting their journey. While both PICS and long COVID are multifaceted and include numerous symptoms and concerns, 3 of the most prevalent ones are brain fog, fatigue and post-exertional malaise, as well as psychological symptoms.

BRAIN FOG
Definition

Different from patient to patient, brain fog is an umbrella term that encompasses a series of cognitive changes including difficulty with problem-solving, reasoning, word-finding, visual-spatial awareness, memory, learning, and attention.[18,19] Cognitive challenges are often described subjectively by patients but can also be measured objectively on examination using screening tools such as the mini-mental state examination, Montreal cognitive assessment, Saint Louis Missouri mental status examination, Mini-Cog, short test of mental status, or repeatable battery for the assessment of neuropsychological status (RBANS).[7,18,19] Subjectively, patients describe feeling "foggy" or "fuzzy," commonly reporting losing their train of thought or forgetting what task they had aimed to complete. In severe cases, some have reported getting lost on commonly driven routes, suffering from aphasia, or failing to remember how to perform tasks that were once routine for them.

Although recognized as a possible sequela of both critical illness and/or a COVID-19 infection, the pathophysiology in each case remains poorly understood. In terms of PASC, some research indicates that COVID-19 may cause inflammation in the brain that precipitates these symptoms[20] while in PICS a similar mechanism has also been explored, but not validated.[4] Most recently, research has been published which indicates that some PASC symptoms, such as brain fog, may be explained by serotonin reduction.[21] While on the other hand, other potential theories around causative factors of brain fog in PICS include fluctuations in glucose, delirium, or in-hospital stress.[22]

Prevalence

Despite the enigmatic biological mechanisms behind brain fog, the prevalence of brain fog reported in PASC and PICS remains high. Anecdotally, cognitive challenges are amongst the most widely reported symptoms in the Survivorship Program. Although the research is limited, it also supports this finding objectively. A systematic review estimating the frequency of persistent symptoms after acute COVID-19 infection identified that about 24% of patients continued to report difficulty concentrating, 19%, reported memory issues and about 18% reported cognitive impairment.[23] Other meta-analyses indicate that the prevalence of cognitive challenges in PASC patients may range from 7.2% to 59.2%.[19]

Similarly, cognitive challenges are amongst the most reported symptoms in after critically ill patients. A 2018 prospective cohort study found that 38% of subjects had cognitive impairment at 3-month follow-up and 33% had cognitive impairment at 12-month follow-up as measured by RBANS. Additionally, a mixed methods pilot investigation conducted by Maley and colleagues[24] revealed that about half of critical illness survivors interviewed reported memory and problem-solving as worse at 6 to 12 months after critical illness.

Treatment

As is the case with the majority of PASC and PICS symptoms, the treatment plan for cognitive challenges related to either etiology are largely rehabilitative in nature. Interestingly, the symptomology of brain fog is similar to that of concussion or traumatic brain injury, and thus established treatment protocols for these disease processes are often utilized in the management of brain fog.[18] This approach involves a structured and individualized plan tailored to the patient's symptoms, lifestyle, and goals, the cornerstones of which involve energy management and memory and organization techniques.[18]

In the Survivorship Program, cognitive rehabilitation is often initiated through a referral with occupational therapy or neuropsychiatry, although in severe cases, a consultation with cognitive neurology may be warranted. Depending on the patient's symptoms, interventions such as frequent mental breaks, taking notes or utilizing electronic reminders, and journaling are often recommended. Additionally, proper sleep hygiene, reduction of screen time, and stress management are integral to the treatment plan.[18]

In the realm of stress management, a unique intervention offered to all patients in the Survivorship Program is a breathing and wellness program, teaching participants yogic breathing and mediation, both of which are evidence-based to support a plethora of mental and physical stressors, including cognitive performance.[25] In follow-up with patients, many report this intervention, if continued consistently, to be powerful to their mental clarity and reduction in brain fog and other symptoms.

PHYSICAL FATIGUE AND POST-EXERTIONAL MALAISE
Definition

There are many different types of fatigue and many different contributing factors.[26,27] The word fatigue is an often-used blanket term to describe different concerns. It is up to clinicians to evaluate the underlying issues and disease processes by using assessments that can consist of aerobic capacity, breathing pattern, perceived fatigue levels, functional capacity, and orthostatic intolerance. These tests can be done through different evaluations including 6-minute walking test, 10-minute standing test, tilt table test, Duke Activity Status Index, Fatigue Severity Scale, DePaul Symptom Questionnaire, and the Dyspnea Scale. These assessments correlate with patient complaints of shortness of breath with exercise and talking, tiredness, activity intolerance, and post-exertional malaise with activity. While difficult to describe, fatigue can be life altering for patients and should be taken seriously.[26]

Prevalence

It is generally understood that fatigue is one of the most prevalent long COVID symptoms,[28] with 1 meta-analysis finding that 32% of individuals who were 12 or more weeks past their COVID-19 diagnosis were experiencing fatigue.[29] Another study found that long COVID patients experiencing fatigue to be as high as 82%.[15] Similarly to long COVID, PICS has high rates of fatigue with studies citing between 24% and 70% of patients endorsing this symptom.[4] Regardless of the variable statistics, fatigue remains a prominent symptom of both long COVID and PICS and is arguably the most widely represented symptom in the Survivorship Program.

Treatment

Physical therapy can be leveraged for the treatment of fatigue. Therefore, in the Survivorship Program, the first-line referral for patients reporting fatigue is to this discipline. With previous experience in treating post-exertional malaise, chronic fatigue, and PICS, physical therapists have a deep knowledge base related to these conditions and others that present under the fatigue umbrella. Knowledgeable providers mix patient education with active treatment. Active treatment can include diaphragmatic breathing, coordinating movement patterns with breathing, inspiratory muscle training, stretching, strengthening, and supervised aerobic conditioning. This is often supplemented by a referral to the yogic breathing and wellness program. Patient education also includes symptom management, activity pacing, energy conservation strategies, and perceived exertion scales. It should also be noted that physical exertion can impact symptom flares and should be under the supervision of providers who understand the long COVID or PICS process.[15]

PSYCHOLOGICAL SYMPTOMS
Definition

Psychological symptoms, such as anxiety, depression, and post-traumatic stress, are often experienced by patients with PICS[4,6,30] and long COVID.[30–32] Anxiety is a persistent mental health disorder when an individual's fear is out of proportion to a perceived threat that will inhibit an individual's daily functioning resulting in behavioral disturbances. Individuals who have an anxiety disorder exhibit anxiousness, fear, and avoidance due to an internal threat to oneself or external threats in their environment. It is important to consider that fear is an appropriate reaction to a perceived threat, whereas anxiety is a state of anxiousness concerning future perceived threats.[33]

Anxiety will often co-occur with major depressive disorder, more commonly known as depression.[33,34] Depression is characterized by persistent sadness, poor appetite, loss of interest and/or pleasure, low energy, poor sleep, and at times suicidal ideations that disrupts daily activities and psychosocial functioning for most of the day, every day, for at least 2 weeks.[34–36] Those diagnosed with long COVID or PICS may experience challenges to their identity and changes in their social role,[37] resulting in anxiety and depression. Potential stressors that can exacerbate one's psychosocial symptoms of long COVID or PICS are the loss of work, the emotional strain of quarantine and isolation, the concern for transmitting COVID-19 or other communicable disease, the high perceived life threat, and the social stigmatization of having been diagnosed with COVID-19 or another disease, all of which is commonly reported in the Survivorship Program.[30]

Post-traumatic stress disorder (PTSD) is caused by the aftereffects from a traumatic event that can cause physical, emotional, spiritual, or psychological harm. Symptoms of PTSD include reliving upsetting memories, nightmares, flashbacks, physical reactions, such as changes in heart rate and blood pressure after re-exposure from a traumatic trigger, or emotional distress.[32] Symptoms of PTSD tend to evolve over time and tend to increase over time[32] after an upsetting event, such as an ICU stay due to COVID-19 or other critical illness.

Prevalence

Over the course of the COVID-19 pandemic, evidence continues to grow that those who are infected with COVID-19 infection have a greater risk of developing mental health and psychological symptoms.[31,32,37] One study found that nearly 34% of people who tested positive for COVID-19 were then diagnosed with either a neurologic or psychiatric diagnosis within the following 6 months.[31] These findings are multifactorial in nature with the prevalence of developing psychological symptoms following a diagnosis of COVID-19 due to the virus itself, as well as the psychological impacts of infection.[37]

The prevalence of the psychosocial limitations (anxiety, depression, and post-traumatic stress) of long COVID are varied. Cenat and colleagues[38] conducted a systemic review to estimate the prevalence of these psychosocial limitations. The prevalence of depression in those with long COVID was nearly 16%, the prevalence of anxiety was 15%, and the prevalence of post-traumatic stress was 22%.[38] All groups diagnosed with COVID- 19, regardless of gender, age, and region, were affected by mental health limitations, with a higher prevalence of depression, anxiety, and post-traumatic stress.

In the realm of critical illness, it is estimated that up to 30% of all critical care survivors diagnosed with COVID-19 will develop PTSD.[39] Additional research indicates that a third of patients report the presence of anxiety and depression after their critical illness with COVID-19.[40] Similarly in the general PICS population, research by Schwitzer and colleagues[41] suggests that as many as 62% of patients endorse anxiety, 36% endorse depression, and 39% endorse PTSD after their ICU stay.

Treatment

Interdisciplinary treatment that focuses on long-term rehabilitation, especially for the psychosocial symptoms of anxiety, depression, and PTSD is necessary for recovery.[30] The COVID-19 pandemic can be classified as a mass casualty incident. As it is difficult to detect and treat psychosocial symptoms and limitations from a mass casualty incident,[39] it is important to develop creative solutions to treatments. The Survivorship Program at BIDMC includes interventions aimed at diagnosing and treating these psychosocial and mental health limitations. Interdisciplinary health care members in the Survivorship Program who focus on the psychosocial limitations from long COVID and PICS include social workers, psychiatrists, and nurses, among others. Additionally, the Survivorship Program keeps those who suffer from long COVID and/or PICS and their loved ones up to date through a quarterly long COVID newsletter along with appropriate follow-up appointments. There are also support groups available for those who have psychosocial symptoms, a behavioral health guide resource, and a personalized digital wellness application program that individuals can use intermittently as needed.[42]

SUMMARY

As the pandemic has progressed, it has become clear that COVID-19 continues to have an effect on many patients well beyond their acute illness. The novel virus has shined a spotlight on many areas of medicine and has brought more attention to the risks for

PICS in both patients with COVID-19 infections, and other patient populations. Currently, both long COVID and PICS are being treated through symptom management rather than treatment of underlying causes. Without formal diagnostic testing or objective criteria, many patients are dismissed by their providers, as well as others, including friends, family, and employers.[43] Keeping this in mind, care should be taken to assess for physical and mental fatigue as well as mental health difficulties in patient populations who are at risk for these illnesses. It is important to encourage active listening and validation of patient symptoms for all providers involved in the care of these patients. Additionally, it is the responsibility of health care clinicians to continue to grow long COVID and PICS survivorships programs to achieve optimal care for this population as coordinated, multidisciplinary care is integral to best outcomes. Further research, funding, and attention are needed to appropriately diagnose and treat long COVID and PICS as well as understand the underlying pathophysiology of both, so the care for this patient population is more optimal and quality of life is improved.

CLINICS CARE POINTS

- In the aftermath of the COVID-19 pandemic, there are unprecedented numbers of patients who continue to suffer with long COVID and/or PICS.
- Nurses must work to recognize and validate symptoms of these intersecting disease processes and advocate for treatment.
- Ongoing, multidisciplinary coordinated care is integral for this patient population.
- Advocacy for the prioritization of research and expansion of survivorship programs is critical to the long-term outcomes of this patient population.

DISCLOSURE

None reported by the authors.

REFERENCES

1. Massachusetts Department of Public Health. Archive of COVID-19 Cases (2020-2021) | Mass.gov. www.mass.gov. https://www.mass.gov/info-details/archive-of-covid-19-cases-2020-2021#april-2020.
2. O'Donoghue SC, Donovan B, Anderson J, et al. Doubling intensive care unit capacity by surging onto medical-surgical units during the COVID-19 pandemic. Dimens Crit Care Nurs 2021;40(6):345–54.
3. Weidman K, LaFond E, Hoffman KL, et al. Post–intensive care unit syndrome in a cohort of COVID-19 survivors in new york city. Annals of the American Thoracic Society 2022;19(7):1158–68.
4. Hiser S, Fatima A, Ali M, et al. Post-intensive care syndrome (PICS): recent updates. Journal of Intensive Care 2023;11(1). https://doi.org/10.1186/s40560-023-00670-7.
5. Needham DM, Davidson J, Cohen H, et al. Improving long-term outcomes after discharge from intensive care unit. Crit Care Med 2012;40(2):502–9.
6. Eaton TL, Lewis A, Donovan HS, et al. Examining the needs of survivors of critical illness through the lens of palliative care: a qualitative study of survivor experiences. Intensive Crit Care Nurs 2022;75:103362.

7. Marra A, Pandharipande PP, Girard TD, et al. Co-occurrence of post-intensive care syndrome problems among 406 survivors of critical illness. Crit Care Med 2018;46(9):1393–401.

8. Heesakkers H, van der Hoeven JG, Corsten S, et al. Clinical outcomes among patients with 1-year survival following intensive care unit treatment for COVID-19. JAMA 2022;327(6):559.

9. Rapin A, Boyer F, Mourvillier B, et al. Post-intensive care syndrome prevalence six months after critical covid-19: comparison between first and second waves. J Rehabil Med 2022;54:jrm00339.

10. Huggins EL, Bloom SL, Stollings JL, et al. A clinic model: post-intensive care syndrome and post-intensive care syndrome-family. AACN Adv Crit Care 2016;27(2):204–11.

11. El-Sadr WM, Vasan A, El-Mohandes A. Facing the new covid-19 reality. N Engl J Med 2023;388(5):385–7.

12. Cutler DM. The costs of long COVID. JAMA Health Forum 2022;3(5):e221809.

13. Davis HE, McCorkell L, Vogel JM, et al. Long COVID: major findings, mechanisms and recommendations. Nat Rev Microbiol 2023;21(3):1–14.

14. CDC. Long COVID - Household Pulse Survey - COVID-19. www.cdc.gov. Published July 19, 2022. https://www.cdc.gov/nchs/covid19/pulse/long-covid.htm.

15. Tabacof L, Tosto-Mancuso J, Wood J, et al. Post-acute COVID-19 syndrome negatively impacts physical function, cognitive function, health-related quality of life, and participation. Am J Phys Med Rehabil 2022;101(1):48–52.

16. Merad M, Blish CA, Sallusto F, et al. The immunology and immunopathology of COVID-19. Science 2022;375(6585):1122–7.

17. Thaweethai T, Jolley SE, Karlson EW, et al. Development of a definition of postacute sequelae of SARS-CoV-2 infection. JAMA 2023;329(22). https://doi.org/10.1001/jama.2023.8823.

18. Fine JS, Ambrose AF, Didehbani N, et al. Multi-disciplinary collaborative consensus guidance statement on the assessment and treatment of cognitive symptoms in patients with post-acute sequelae of SARS-CoV-2 infection (PASC). PM&R 2022;14(1):96–111.

19. Quan M, Wang X, Gong M, et al. Post-COVID cognitive dysfunction: current status and research recommendations for high risk population. Lancet 2023;38:100836.

20. Fernández-Castañeda A, Lu P, Geraghty AC, et al. Mild respiratory COVID can cause multi-lineage neural cell and myelin dysregulation. Cell 2022;185(14):2452–68.e16.

21. Wong AC, Devason AS, Umana IC, et al. Serotonin reduction in post-acute sequelae of viral infection. Cell 2023;186(22). https://doi.org/10.1016/j.cell.2023.09.013.

22. Inoue S, Hatakeyama J, Kondo Y, et al. Post-intensive care syndrome: its pathophysiology, prevention, and Future Directions. Acute Medicine & Surgery 2019;6(3):233–46.

23. Groff D, Sun A, Ssentongo AE, et al. Short-term and long-term rates of postacute sequelae of SARS-CoV-2 infection: a systematic review. JAMA Netw Open 2021;4(10):e2128568.

24. Maley JH, Brewster I, Mayoral I, et al. Resilience in survivors of critical illness in the context of the survivors' experience and recovery. Annals of the American Thoracic Society 2016;13(8):1351–60.

25. Rain M, Subramaniam B, Avti P, et al. Can yogic breathing techniques like simha kriya and isha kriya regulate COVID-19-related stress? Front Psychol 2021;12. https://doi.org/10.3389/fpsyg.2021.635816.

26. Kuppuswamy A. The fatigue conundrum. Brain 2017;140(8):2240–5.

27. Twomey R, DeMars J, Franklin K, et al. Chronic fatigue and postexertional malaise in people living with long COVID: an observational study. Phys Ther 2022;102(4). https://doi.org/10.1093/ptj/pzac005.
28. Yong SJ. Long COVID or post-COVID-19 syndrome: putative pathophysiology, risk factors, and treatments. Infectious Diseases 2021;53(10):1–18.
29. Ceban F, Ling S, Lui LMW, et al. Fatigue and cognitive impairment in post-COVID-19 syndrome: a systematic review and meta-analysis. Brain Behav Immun 2021; 101. https://doi.org/10.1016/j.bbi.2021.12.020.
30. Higgins V, Sohaei D, Diamandis EP, et al. COVID-19: from an acute to chronic disease? potential long-term health consequences. Crit Rev Clin Lab Sci 2020;58(5):1–23.
31. Taquet M, Geddes JR, Husain M, et al. 6-month neurological and psychiatric outcomes in 236 379 survivors of COVID-19: a retrospective cohort study using electronic health records. Lancet Psychiatr 2021;8(5). https://doi.org/10.1016/S2215-0366(21)00084-5.
32. Houben-Wilke S, Goërtz YM, Delbressine JM, et al. The impact of long COVID-19 on mental health: observational 6-month follow-up study. JMIR Mental Health 2022;9(2):e33704.
33. Craske MG, Stein MB. Anxiety. Lancet 2016;388(10063):3048–59.
34. Li Z, Ruan M, Chen J, et al. Major depressive disorder: advances in neuroscience research and translational applications. Neurosci Bull 2021;37(6). https://doi.org/10.1007/s12264-021-00638-3.
35. World Health Organization. Mental Disorders. World Health Organization. Published June 8, 2022. https://www.who.int/news-room/fact-sheets/detail/mental-disorders.
36. Spence NJ, Russell D, Bouldin ED, et al. Getting back to normal? Identity and role disruptions among adults with Long COVID. Sociol Health Illness 2023;45(4). https://doi.org/10.1111/1467-9566.13628.
37. Stucke J, Maxwell E, House J. Long Covid 2: supporting the mental and physical needs of patients. Nursing Times. Published June 27, 2022. https://www.nursingtimes.net/clinical-archive/long-term-conditions/long-covid-2-supporting-the-mental-and-physical-needs-of-patients-27-06-2022/.
38. Cénat JM, Blais-Rochette C, Kokou-Kpolou CK, et al. Prevalence of symptoms of depression, anxiety, insomnia, posttraumatic stress disorder, and psychological distress among populations affected by the COVID-19 pandemic: a systematic review and meta-analysis. Psychiatr Res 2021;295:113599.
39. Greene T, El-Leithy S, Billings J, et al. Anticipating PTSD in severe COVID survivors: the case for screen-and-treat. Eur J Psychotraumatol 2022;13(1). https://doi.org/10.1080/20008198.2021.1959707.
40. Larsson IM, Hultström M, Miklós L, et al. Poor long-term recovery after critical COVID-19 during 12 months longitudinal follow-up. Intensive Crit Care Nurs 2023;74(103311):103311.
41. Schwitzer E, Schwab K, Brinkman L, et al. Survival ≠ recovery. CHEST Critical Care 2023;1(1):100003.
42. Critical Illness and COVID-19 Survivorship Program. www.bidmc.org. https://www.bidmc.org/centers-and-departments/pulmonary-critical-care-and-sleep-medicine/services-and-programs/critical-illness-survivorship-program.
43. McManimen S, McClellan D, Stoothoff J, et al. Dismissing chronic illness: a qualitative analysis of negative health care experiences. Health Care Women Int 2019; 40(3):241–58.

The Impact of Coronavirus Disease 2019 on Nursing Education
Evidence, Experience, and Lessons Learned

Lisa Connelly, DNP, RN[a], Casey Cunha, DNP, RN, CNP[a],
Karen Wholey, MSN, RN[a],
Justin H. DiLibero, DNP, APRN, CCRN, ACCNS-AG, FCNS[b],*

KEYWORDS

- Nursing education • Practice-readiness • Post-pandemic challenges
- Nursing workforce • Experience-complexity gap • Remote learning

KEY POINTS

The coronavirus disease 2019 pandemic brought both challenges and opportunities to academic nursing education including

- A rapid shift to remote learning: The pandemic required a rapid shift in nursing education to remote learning. While this created significant challenges during the early pandemic, it also creates new opportunities for educators and students as we move into the post-pandemic era.
- Adaptation and integration of technology: The adaptation and integration of clinical and educational technology in nursing education and clinical practice were critical to addressing challenges experienced during the pandemic and create new opportunities in the post-pandemic era. This article will emphasize the ways in which technology has become an invaluable tool in a post-pandemic world.
- Challenges in clinical education: The pandemic imposed unique challenges in clinical education including the inability to complete clinical rotations and the implications for skill development necessary for practice.
- The psychological toll of stress and burnout: The psychological impact of the pandemic on nursing students, faculty, and professionals, is often under-recognized. This article will delve into the challenges of stress and burnout within the context of critical care nursing and academic nursing education.
- Nursing shortage and workforce factors: Although nursing workforce challenges existed before the pandemic, the pandemic intensified the nursing shortage and the influence of workforce dynamics on nursing education, particularly the demand for critical care nurses.

[a] Rhode Island College, Fogarty Life Science Building, Room 158, 600 Mount Pleasant Avenue, Providence, RI 02908, USA; [b] Rhode Island College, Onanian School of Nursing, 600 Mount Pleasant Avenue, Providence, RI 02908, USA
* Corresponding author.
E-mail address: jdilibero@ric.edu

Crit Care Nurs Clin N Am 36 (2024) 437–449
https://doi.org/10.1016/j.cnc.2023.12.001
0899-5885/24/© 2023 Elsevier Inc. All rights reserved.
ccnursing.theclinics.com

INTRODUCTION

The coronavirus disease 2019 (COVID-19) pandemic has left a lasting mark on the health care system, triggering a series of challenges that reverberated across the industry. These challenges evolved over the course of time, from the emergence of the novel coronavirus to the post-pandemic era. During the early pandemic, health care facilities grappled with issues such as the need to meet the demands of an unprecedented surge in patient volume, overwhelming both physical resources and personnel capacity.[1] This surge placed immense pressure on clinicians who found themselves grappling with a dearth of knowledge regarding the pathophysiology, pharmacologic treatments, evidence-based patient management strategies, and infection control measures.[2–4] This impacted all facets of the health care system, especially critical care areas where the need for rapid adaptations to patient care was crucial.

While the needs of the clinical setting were paramount, academic nursing education, integral to shaping the next generation of professional nurses, found itself in a parallel struggle. The pandemic necessitated an abrupt shift to remote learning, creating hurdles in clinical education and contributing to student stress and disengagement.[5]

However intense the challenges of the early pandemic, the post-pandemic era brings a new set of challenges and opportunities for nursing practice and education. The retirement of the baby boomer generation and the departure of experienced nurses from the bedside, compounded by the pandemic's impact, have created a demand for nursing positions that outpaces the graduation of new nurses.[6] Notably, many new nurses are entering the workforce directly into highly specialized areas, including critical care. These nurses find themselves in a rapidly evolving health care landscape characterized by increasingly complex systems and fewer experienced mentors to guide them, giving rise to what is known as the 'experience-complexity gap.'[7] This gap leads to increased stress levels fueling a vicious cycle of burnout and turnover.[8–10] Solving these challenges demands a collaborative effort between academic and clinical settings to address the structural causes of burnout and turnover.

In the pages that follow, this article will delve into the multifaceted implications of the COVID-19 pandemic on nursing education and related implications for critical care nursing. The topics explored in the following sections include the rapid shift to remote learning, challenges in clinical education, the psychological toll of stress and burnout, ethical dilemmas in care provision, adaptation and integration of clinical and educational technology, pandemic-specific alterations to the nursing curriculum, and the invaluable lessons drawn from this unprecedented crisis. Understanding the evolving dynamics of the pandemic is not only vital for informing nursing educators and practicing nurses alike. It presents an opportunity for each of us, individually and collectively, to contribute to a more ideal future.

SHIFT TO ONLINE LEARNING

The COVID-19 pandemic triggered a significant shift in nursing education, requiring schools and universities worldwide to transition to online learning.[11–13] Given the hands-on nature of the profession, this transition presented both opportunities and challenges for nursing students, educators, and institutions.

Nursing education, comprised of didactic (classroom) and clinical learning, traditionally places a strong emphasis on experiential learning in clinical settings, where students develop essential skills through direct practice experiences. Didactic education can be delivered through in-person or online modalities, depending upon the program's design. However, programs that primarily utilized in-person instruction were required to transition to online or distance learning when the pandemic began. Importantly, quality remote and online education requires appropriate infrastructure, intentional design, and skilled facilitation by a knowledgeable educator trained in this pedagogy. However, during the pandemic, the shift to remote and online courses often occurred among courses not designed or intended for this modality, in the absence of essential technology and infrastructure, and taught by faculty without training or experience in this area.[14] This transition also introduced technological challenges for students such as limited access to high-speed Internet.[11,15,16] Collectively, the rapid shift to online didactic education posed challenges for students and faculty alike.

In addition to didactic instruction, clinical placements play a crucial role in nursing education, allowing students to apply theoretic knowledge in real-word health care settings. Even before the pandemic, students faced difficulties mastering competence such as delegation, prioritization, time management, and clinical decision-making, underscoring the need for increased hands-on learning.[17] These challenges were exacerbated by the pandemic as nursing programs faced disruptions and curriculum alterations, leaving students and new nurses with heightened stress levels and feelings of unpreparedness.[18]

At the onset of the pandemic, clinical placements were temporarily suspended; however, as more information about the virus became available and demand for support in health care facilities grew, clinical sites gradually began allowing students to return to clinical. During this time, clinical placements were limited, resulting in a continued shortage of practical learning opportunities.

Pre-pandemic, research has demonstrated the advantages of simulation and supporting its integration into nursing curricula to enhance students' skills and readiness for practice.[19] For these reasons, when faced with limited clinical placements, many programs turned to simulation and virtual laboratories as a replacement for lost clinical time.[18] These platforms offered a controlled environment for students to practice skills, often incorporating computer-generated patient scenarios and virtual reality technology.

In 2014, the National Council of State Boards of Nursing (NCSBN) published a study supporting the replacement of up to 50% traditional clinical hours with high-fidelity simulation experiences, producing similar end-of-program outcomes and graduate preparedness.[20] Despite the NCSBN's support for the use of simulation in place of a portion of traditional clinical hours, the specific clinical requirements are determined by individual's state's boards of nursing, which have not all adopted this recommendation. However, some states that did not adopt the NCSBN recommendation as a standard practice did temporarily increase the allowable simulation hours during the pandemic. For example, California issued an executive order temporarily allowing up to 50% of clinical time to be allocated to simulation.[21]

While these strategies offered valuable learning experiences, they do not fully replicate the complexity and unpredictability of real-life patient interactions, and some faculty have questioned the level of student preparedness when real-life patient interactions are limited.[22] The shift to online learning also necessitated the adaptation of assessment methods in nursing education. Traditionally, assessments involved observations of students in the practice settings. With limited access to clinical placements, educators had to explore alternative assessment strategies, such as evaluating students' demonstrations of assessment skills using video communication platforms and assessments of virtual simulation experiences.

FACULTY SUPPORT AND TRAINING

Amid the COVID-19 pandemic, nursing faculty faced the urgent need to adapt their teaching methodologies, transitioning from traditional in-person instruction to online learning. Many faculty members required substantial support during this transition, as educational institutions across the globe swiftly shifted to remote learning to ensure the safety of students, staff, and faculty. This move to online teaching presented a multitude of challenges for faculty members who were not accustomed to delivering their courses through digital platforms.

Common challenges faced by faculty during this transition included

Technical proficiency: Many faculty members lacked familiarity with online teaching tools and platforms, necessitating training and support to navigate virtual classrooms, video conferencing tools, learning management systems (LMSs), and other educational technologies.[14,23]

Course redesign: Converting traditional in-person courses into effective online formats required careful consideration and redesign. Faculty required assistance restructuring their course materials, assessments, and activities to align with online learning environments.

Pedagogical guidance: Effective online teaching requires distinct instructional strategies and approaches compared to face-to-face teaching. Faculty required guidance on engaging students effectively, promoting active learning, and sustaining student motivation in a virtual setting.

Accessibility and inclusivity: Ensuring that online courses are accessible to all students, including those with disabilities or limited access to technology, was a concern for faculty. They needed support in making their courses inclusive and accommodating diverse learning needs.

Time management: Transitioning to online teaching demanded additional time and effort from faculty, especially those unacquainted with online instruction. Balancing teaching responsibilities with other demands proved to be a significant challenge.

To address these challenges, many educational institutions provided faculty with professional development opportunities, workshops, and resources to enhance their online teaching skills. They also offered support such as instructional designers, technology specialists, and learning technology teams to assist faculty in effectively adapting their courses. Collaborative online platforms and communities emerged, enabling faculty to exchange best practices, share resources, and seek advice from peers experienced in online teaching. The collective efforts and support from the educational community helped many faculty members successfully transition to online teaching during the COVID-19 pandemic.[23]

While the abrupt shift certainly brought challenges, it also provided opportunities for innovation and creativity. For example, the shift to virtual platforms allowed real-time interaction with students and peers despite the need for remote instruction. These platforms served various purposes, from hosting live sessions to conducting office hours, advising, and discussing course-related matters.

Moreover, faculty leveraged LMSs to organize and centralize course materials, assignments, quizzes, and discussions. The use of discussion boards in courses increased, and examinations were formatted for secure administration through these platforms. Faculty also became proficient in delivering these assessments through secure platforms to maintain academic integrity. Finally, recognizing the challenges faced by students during the pandemic, such as Internet connectivity issues, home environments, personal health concerns, and emotional influence, many faculty members adapted to provide essential support and foster an inclusive learning environment.

PSYCHOLOGICAL IMPACT ON NURSING STUDENTS

Nursing students have long struggled with high levels of anxiety stemming from the inherent stressors associated with their academic pursuits, challenging course materials, and the physical and emotional demands of their studies.[24] However, the onset of the COVID-19 pandemic introduced a novel and heightened array of challenges, substantially exacerbating the levels of anxiety and stress typically experienced by nursing students. The pervasive fear surrounding the pandemic and its repercussions played a pivotal role in intensifying the risk of concurrent anxiety and depression among students.[25] Students were worried about the progression of the pandemic and the implications for their own well-being as well as that of their families. The risk of disease transmission to their family and friends created additional stress. Notably, students were often more worried about transmission to their loved ones rather than their own exposure to the virus.[26] Furthermore, the uncertain nature associated with the evolving pandemic's impact within the health care workforce contributed significantly to their mental pressure and concerns.[11] Moreover, exposure to media reports on the impact of the COVID-19 on the nursing and health care workforce and the growing issue of burnout were associated with increased psychological distress among aspiring graduates.[25]

Increasing demands in students' personal and professional lives resulted in decreased available time for studying contributing negatively to academic performance. The sudden disruption of coursework, restrictions on community activities, and the abrupt shift to online learning platforms left students feeling overwhelmed. The most important contributors to anxiety during this time included a sudden shift to remote learning, technological challenges for both students and staff, and perceived loss of support mechanisms secondary to feeling isolated from peers.[15] Notably, student's perception of their family's financial vulnerability was an important predictor for higher rates of anxiety and depression."[25] In addition, students faced alarming rates of graduation delays (31%) and loss of internships (40%), factors found to increase mental anguish.[11]

The enforced social isolation often required students to be away from family, friends, and peers. Prolonged quarantine was associated with elevated stress, emotional responses, anxiety, and depression.[25] Additionally, students who were unable to maintain their previous level of physical activity were more likely to experience worsened mental health.[25] Sleep disturbances related to COVID-19 fears and compromised physiologic needs were linked to worsened levels of mental health and a desire to withdraw from nursing programs.[24,25] Unfortunately, resources for mental health support during this period were limited, primarily due to a lack of clinician availability, the transition to telehealth services, or restricted access to school-based programs.

CHALLENGES IN CLINICAL EDUCATION
Student Placement

Numerous ethical considerations emerged for nursing students in the context of clinical placements during the COVID-19 pandemic. Nursing students attending clinical placements shared similar fears with more experienced nurses, which were driven by the rapid spread of the virus, limited access to personal protective equipment (PPE), inexperience handling patient loss, and a profound sense of uncertainty regarding the future.

Nursing students expressed hesitancy in receiving the COVID-19 vaccine, required for clinical placements, due to uncertainties about potential long-term side effects associated with the fast-tracked vaccine approval. They grappled with situations involving rapidly deteriorating COVID-19 patients in isolation and the possible delay of treatment associated with donning of PPE. Nursing students faced ethical dilemmas that they may not have encountered before, such as the challenge of triaging patient care amongst limited resources. They had to adapt to environment in which nontraditional methods for making difficult decisions was required, including rationing critical resources to prioritize patients with a higher likelihood of survival.[27]

Additional ethical considerations were linked to students' clinical placements. Although nursing programs historically mandated the number of clinical hours needed for each course, decisions about permitting students to continue in the clinical setting needed to be weighed against the potential risk of contracting the virus. Nursing students also grappled with the fear of potentially transmitting the virus from the clinical site to their family and friends, often leading to feelings of guilt when a close friend or family member tested positive for COVID-19.[28]

Limitations of Clinical Sites

Clinical site limitations were exacerbated by the pandemic, adding to the existing challenges faced by nursing schools. Units were closed to students due to the high number of COVID-19–positive patients and restrictions that prevented students from caring for such patients. This challenging and uncertain environment coupled with limited support from hospitals for clinical placement jeopardized learning outcomes established by nursing programs, as clinical experience is an important component of a nursing program and essential for credentialing.[29]

Hospitals struggled with increased staffing shortages due to the need for nurses to quarantine, making it difficult for units to accommodate nursing students. The high acuity of patient populations further complicated the ability of staff nurses to adequately supervise and mentor students. Staff nurses believed that the responsibility of supervising students should fall to a dedicated charge nurse or nurse preceptor, as staff nurses were overwhelmed with their existing responsibilities.[28] This situation limited the ability to pair students with experienced preceptors.

Safety Concerns for Students During Clinical Rotations/Infection Control Practices

Numerous safety concerns arose for students during their clinical rotations, along with the need for stringent infection control practices. One significant challenge was that patients often were not tested and/or diagnosed with COVID-19 until after students had already provided care. Insufficient PPE was a concern for both hospital staff and students, placing additional strain on academic programs to ensure student safety.[29] This led to concerns about whether students were exposed to risks that they would not have encountered otherwise, potentially jeopardizing their health.

The COVID-19 pandemic brought about a heightened awareness of infection control practices and infection risks associated with patient care. Students with prior clinical experience were better prepared to practice hand hygiene, standard precautions, and donning and doffing of PPE. Hospitals often offered routine testing for staff on-site, but these measures were not always extended to students due to limited availability, as it was considered the responsibility of the school rather than the clinical site.[29]

Reduced Exposure to Diverse Patient Populations and Conditions

Due to restrictions placed on nursing students in the clinical setting, not only were there limitations on the number of patients available, but also reduced exposure to diverse patient populations and conditions. Students, with their limited clinical experience, were unsure of how to interact and care for patients of diverse backgrounds. They questioned whether patients would be comfortable with students providing care to them and about how to communicate effectively with patients, especially given the constraints imposed by PPE.[28] The pandemic highlighted social issues that the students may not have otherwise been aware of, including the limited availability of testing sites, transportation challenges, and a lack of accessible technology such as Internet and computer access, which are essential for individuals to actively participate in their care.[30]

ETHICAL DILEMMAS IN CRITICAL CARE

The COVID-19 pandemic presented numerous ethical dilemmas in critical care settings. Some common ethical challenges faced by health care professionals during this time included the allocation of limited resources, triage decisions, the balance between their duty to care and personal risk, and end-of-life decisions. These ethical dilemmas took an emotional toll, often contributing to moral distress.[2,30]

The rapid progression of the virus led to a substantial increase in patient volume, particularly among the elderly and those with severe illnesses. This surge placed significant strain on the health care system in many countries, causing shortages of critical medical resources such as ventilators and critical care beds. The overwhelming demand exceeded the capacity of health care resources, necessitating the difficult task of rationing medical equipment and interventions.[31]

A review of the literature by Dowling and colleagues[31] on the allocation of scarce medical resources during the COVID-19 pandemic revealed findings that aligned with an opinion paper published in the New England Journal of Medicine.[32] Both groups emphasized the goal of reducing mortality, saving the youngest patients, and saving the greatest number of lives.[31,32] Nurses were faced with the difficult responsibility of conducting conversations about goals of care, resuscitation preferences, and advance directives while considering the emotional toll on patients and their families.

Ethical dilemmas also revolved around patient isolation measures and visitor restrictions implemented to prevent the spread of the virus. While isolation measures were needed to protect patients' health and reduce the spread of COVID-19, they impacted patient's autonomy and psychological well-being.[33] While nurses found ways to facilitate communication between patients and their loved as best as possible while they maintained infection control protocols, they observed an increase in patients' depression and anxiety levels.[33,34] This, in turn, contributed to an increase in nurses experiencing moral distress.[35]

The pandemic brought to light preexisting health disparities, with certain populations being disproportionately affected by COVID-19. Nurses had to confront these inequities and advocate for equitable access to health care services and resources.[35]

CHANGES IN CURRICULUM

The impact of the pandemic spurred educational institutions to recognize the need for curriculum revisions to meet the evolving learning needs of their students. This included the incorporation of content specific to the evolving pandemic.

Integration of Coronavirus Disease 2019–Specific Content

Essential content related to COVID-19 included topics such as acute respiratory distress syndrome, patient proning, the emerging issue of long COVID, COVID transmission dynamics, and the proper utilization of PPE for transmission prevention. Effective methods for integrating this COVID-19–specific content include didactic instruction, case studies, gaming, flipped classrooms, simulations, and alternative teaching approaches, which have demonstrated their effectiveness in facilitating the retention of critical information.[36]

Emphasis on Infection Prevention and Control Measures

Nursing curriculum should place a strong focus on the prevention of virus transmission. This includes an in-depth understanding of current quarantine requirements and the correct use of PPE, all of which are essential to ensuring the safety of nursing students.[28]

Enhanced Focus on Critical Care and Emergency Preparedness

The pandemic offered nurse educators a unique opportunity to showcase their capacity for innovation and adaptability within nursing education, especially when confronted with rapidly changing circumstances.[30] As nursing schools transitioned to online learning and alternative teaching methods, nursing organizations disseminated training modules that specifically addressed pandemic-related topics.

A crucial lesson learned from the pandemic is that both nursing education curricula and clinical practice must incorporate robust emergency preparedness and public health response training. This should include the implementation of emergency mock drills and disaster training exercises.[37]

RECOMMENDATIONS FOR NURSING EDUCATION

Historically nursing education has focused on the accumulation of required clinical hours as a measure of success rather than the demonstration of clinical competence. This approach may be ineffective as competency attainment is less a function of time and more a function of meaningful engagement and the facilitation of learning.[30] To enhance clinical competence, clinical experiences can be woven throughout the curriculum to create an interactive and dynamic learning experience. Such an approach can enhance students' ability to explore the social implications of diseases and their effects on diverse patient populations within the broader health care system, rather than viewing diseases in isolation.[30] Importantly, such approaches de-emphasize the simple accumulation of hours in favor of more dynamic and interconnected learning while enhancing students' development of competence.

Strengthening Virtual Learning Capabilities and Resources

Significant downfalls were associated with remote and online learning during the COVID-19 pandemic. Rapid transitions from traditional in-person classes to online formats posed significant challenges for both students and faculty. Engagement and focus on course content became formidable tasks. Additionally, concerns arose regarding the accessibility of online education, especially among students who lacked reliable Internet access or a dedicated, quiet learning environment at home. The online setting often failed to support meaningful interaction between students and instructors, particularly for those who struggled in virtual learning. Many students benefitted from additional resources and support services offered by educational institutions, which played a pivotal role in their program success.[30]

Enhancing Simulation-Based Training and Debriefing Techniques

Creating appropriate clinical experiences for students can be a complex endeavor, especially when aiming to expose them to diverse patient populations and complex health care scenarios. Virtual and online educational experiences, while not substitutes for in-person clinical experiences, can serve as valuable supplements.[38] Simulation-based training offers students the opportunity to engage in realistic patient scenarios, providing a consistent and controlled environment that aligns with course objectives and enhances clinical learning.[30]

Debriefing, an integral part of simulation-based training, allows students to reflect on their experiences and engage in thoughtful discussions about their strengths and areas in need of improvement.[28] This safe learning environment enables students to develop critical thinking skills and collaborative teamwork while treating complex patient care scenarios.[30]

Prioritizing Mental Health Support Services for Nursing Students

Nursing programs should ensure that students are not only aware of available mental health resources but also of those supporting their overall success, especially during challenging times. The pandemic has highlighted the importance of educators' support, compassion toward students' physical and mental well-being, and flexibility in assignments. Studies have shown that students who received such support exhibited reduced anxiety and stress, enabling them to adapt to difficult circumstances with increased confidence and less self-doubt.[28]

Stress Management and Resilience Training

Students should have access to a variety of resources promoting self-care, stress management techniques, and resilience training. A comprehensive set of resources should be available to help students effectively cope with stress and anxiety, address ethical challenges, and make sound decisions based on the prevailing circumstances and desired outcomes.[28]

Establishing Collaborative Partnerships Between Academic Institutions and Health care Facilities

Looking ahead, enhancing collaborative partnerships between academic institutions and health care facilities is imperative. Hospitals are currently grappling with an unprecedented staffing crisis, resulting in nurses leaving both bedside and the profession altogether. To counter this, the number of graduating students must increase, and more important strategies to retain nurses in the practice setting must be employed. Nurses must be prepared to be adaptable and resilient in the ever-changing health care landscape. Fostering an environment of care and openness between students and mentors and experienced nurses alike in place of a culture of incivility where nurses "eat their young" is critical. This requires the cultivation of a culture based on trust and support, promoting a "sense of belonging," where individuals feel valued, accepted, and integrated.[29]

Continual communication between nursing schools and clinical placement sites is necessary to ensure students are prepared to respond effectively to health care emergencies, such as a pandemic. Strengthening the learning experiences provided at clinical sites is vital to meet all relevant content and competency requirements.[37]

SUMMARY

This article has provided a comprehensive overview of the challenges and adaptations in nursing education during the pandemic and the interconnectedness of challenges in the academic and practice environments. The article sheds light on the significant psychological impact on nursing students and raises the importance of support, training for faculty, and provision of essential technology and infrastructure within nursing education programs to meet student needs. With a shared understanding of the challenges, innovations, and emerging solutions, we will be able to enhance student learning, better bridging the gap between academic learning and the realities of the practice setting necessary to support the needs of the current and future nursing workforce.

CLINICS CARE POINTS

- The pandemic has imparted invaluable lessons on the health care system which have been well documented.[39,40] These include
- The need for preparedness and planning: The importance of comprehensive pandemic response plans has been underscored, emphasizing the need for proactive preparedness.[41]
- The importance of infection control and prevention: Nurses played a pivotal role in implementing infection control measures to safeguard patients and themselves.[42]
- The need for resource management and allocation: Nurses became adept at optimizing limited resources, including PPE and medical supplies. Nurses should be recognized, included, and supported for their essential decision-making roles.[43,44]
- The need for adaptability: Nurses exhibited remarkable adaptability and flexibility in responding to rapidly evolving guidelines, protocols, and treatments.[45]
- The need for emotional support: Recognizing the emotional and psychological stress endured by nurses, the importance of providing support and promoting self-care has become paramount in reducing burnout and maintaining well-being.[46]
- The need for interdisciplinary collaboration: Collaboration among health care professionals, particularly nurses, was highlighted as vital for holistic patient care.[47]
- The need to integrate technology: The accelerated adoption of telehealth and digital solutions has prompted nurses to acquire new skills for remote patient monitoring, virtual consultations, and distance education.[48]
- The need for public health advocacy: Nurses assumed a central role in educating the public about COVID-19, its transmission, prevention, and vaccination, emerging as advocates for public health initiatives.[49]
- The need to address health disparities: The pandemic exposed existing health disparities and the impact of social determinants of health on vulnerable populations, compelling nurses to address these issues to ensure equitable care.[50]
- The need for resilience and professional growth: Nurses demonstrated remarkable resilience, coping with challenges and emerging as even stronger and more skilled health care professionals.[51]
- The need for knowledge sharing and global collaboration: The pandemic highlighted the value of global collaboration and knowledge sharing among health care professionals to effectively respond to global health crises.[52]

DISCLOSURE

None of the authors have any disclosures to report.

REFERENCES

1. Arabi Y, Myatra S, Lobo S. Surging ICU during COVID-19 pandemic: an overview. Curr Opin Crit Care 2022;28(6):638–44.

2. Aydogu A. Ethical dilemmas experienced by nurses while caring for patients during the COVID-19 pandemic: an integrative review of qualitative studies. J Nurs Manag 2022;1–14. https://doi.org/10.1097/MCC.0000000000001001.

3. Guttormson J, Calkins K, McAndrews N, et al. Critical care nurses' experience during the COVID-19 pandemic: a US national survey. Am J Crit Care 2022; 31(2):96–103.

4. Moore D, Dawkins D, Hampton M, et al. Experience of critical care nurses during the early months of the COVID-19 pandemic. Nurs Ethics 2022;29(3):540–51.

5. Lever C, Stanley J, Veenema T. Impact of the COVID-19 pandemic on the future of nursing education. Acad Med 2022;91(35):S82–9.

6. American Association of Colleges of Nursing. Fact sheet: nursing shortage. 2022 Available at: https://www.aacnnursing.org/Portals/0/PDFs/Fact-Sheets/Nursing-Shortage-Factsheet.pdf. Accessed August 29, 2023.

7. Virkstis K, Herleth A, Rewers L. Closing nursing's experience-complexity gap. J Nurs Adm 2019;49(12):580–2.

8. Martin B, Kaminski-Ozturk N, O'Hara C, et al. Examining the impact of the COVID-19 pandemic on burnout and stress among US Nurses. J Nurs Regul 2023; 14(1):4–12.

9. Moss M, Good VS, Gozal D, et al. An official Critical Care Societies Collaborative statement: burnout syndrome in critical care health care professionals: a call for action. Am J Crit Care 2016;25(4):368–76.

10. NSI Nursing Solutions. 2022 National healthcare retention & RN staffing report. NSI Solutions, Inc.; 2022. Available at. https://www.nsinursingsolutions.com/Documents/Library/NSI_National_Health_Care_Retention_Report.pd. Accessed July 6, 2022.

11. Farsi Z, Sajadi S, Afaghi, et al. Explaining the experience of nursing administrators, educators and students about education process in the covid-19 pandemic: a qualitative study. BMC Nurs 2021;20(1):2–13.

12. Flølo T, Gjeilo K, Anderson J, Andersen JR, et al. The impact of educational concerns and satisfaction on baccalaureate nursing students' distress and quality of life during the COVID-19 pandemic: a cross-sectional study. BMC Nurs 2022; 21(1):185.

13. Molefe L, Mobunda N. Online teaching and learning: experiences of students in a nursing college during the onset of COVID-19. Curationis 2022;45(1):e1–10.

14. Nabolsi M, Abu-Moghli F, Khalaf I, et al. Nursing faculty experience with distance education during COVID-19 crisis: a qualitative study. J Prof Nurs 2021;37(5): 828–35.

15. Wallace S, Schuler M, Kaulback M, et al. Nursing student experience of remote learning during the COVID-19 pandemic. Nurs Forum 2021;56(3):612–8.

16. Olum R, Atulinda L, Kigozi E, et al. Medical education and e-learning during COVID-19 Pandemic: awareness, attitudes, preferences, and barriers among undergraduate medicine and nursing students at Makerere University, Uganda. J Med Educ Curricu Dev 2020;7. https://doi.org/10.1111/nuf.12568.

17. Casey K, Fink R, Jaynes C, et al. Readiness for practice: the senior practicum experience. J Nurs Educ 2011;50(11):646–52.

18. Lanahan M, Montalvo B, Cohn T. The perception of preparedness in undergraduate nursing students during COVID-19. J Prof Nurs 2022;42:111–21.

19. Hustad J, Johannesen B, Fossum M, et al. Nursing students' transfer of learning outcomes from simulation-based training to clinical practice: a focus-group study. BMC Nurs 2019;8(18):53.

20. Hayden J, Smiley R, Alexander M, et al. The NCSBN national simulation study: a longitudinal study replacing clinical hours with simulation in prelicensure nursing education. J Nurs Regul 2014;5(2):S3–40.

21. Kirchmeyer K. Memorandum: Guidance on waiver of restrictions on nursing student clinical hours under DCA waiver DCA-20-30. 2020. Retrieved September 1, 2023. Available at: https://www.dca.ca.gov/licensees/clinical_hours_guidance.pdf.

22. Konrad S, Fitzgerald A, Deckers C. Nursing fundamentals: supporting clinical competency online during the COVID-19 pandemic. Teach Learn Nurs 2021; 16(1):53–6.

23. Wilson J, Hensley A, Culp-Roche A, et al. Transitioning to teaching online during the COVID-19 pandemic. Sage Open Nurse 2021;7. https://doi.org/10.1177/23779608211026137.

24. Tanji F, Kodama Y. Presence of psychological distress and associated factors in nursing students during the COVID-19 pandemic: a cross-sectional study. Int J Environ Res Publ Health 2021;18(19):1–10.

25. Li D, Zou L, Zhang Z, et al. The psychological effect of COVID-19 on home-quarantined nursing students in China. Front Psychiatr 2021;12. https://doi.org/10.3389/fpsyt.2021.652296.

26. Barrett D. Impact of COVID-19 on nursing students: what does the evidence tell us? Evid Base Nurs 2022;25(2):37–8.

27. Palacios-Ceña D, Velarde-García JF, Espejo MM, et al. Ethical challenges during the COVID-19 pandemic: perspectives of nursing students. Nurs Ethics 2021; 29(2). https://doi.org/10.1177/09697330211030676. 096973302110306.

28. Dziurka M, Machul M, Ozdoba P, et al. Clinical training during the COVID-19 pandemic: experiences of nursing students and implications for education. Int J Environ Res Publ Health 2022;19(10):6352.

29. Ulenaers D, Grosemans J, Schrooten W, et al. Clinical placement experience of nursing students during the COVID-19 Pandemic: a cross-sectional study. Nurse Educ Today 2021;99(1):104746.

30. Weberg D, Chan G, Dickow M. Disrupting nursing education in light of COVID-19. OJIN: Online J Issues Nurs 2021;26(1). https://doi.org/10.3912/ojin.vol26no01man04.

31. Dowling A, Lane H, Haines T. Community preferences for the allocation of scarce healthcare resources during the COVID-19 pandemic: a review of the literature. Publ Health 2022;209:75–81.

32. Lenton A, Blair I, Hastie R. The influence of social categories and patient responsibility on health care allocation decisions: bias or fairness? Basic Appl Soc Psychol 2006;28(1):27–36.

33. Lavasseur A. Effect of social isolation on long-term care resident with dementia and depression during the COVID-19 pandemic. Geriatr Nurs 2021;42(3):780–1.

34. Gordon C, Thompson A. The use of personal protective equipment during the COVID-19 Pandemic. Br J Nurs 2020;29(13):748–52.

35. Jia Y, Chen O, Xiao Z, et al. Nurses' ethical challenges caring for people with COVID-19: a qualitative study. Nurs Ethics 2021;28(1):33–45.

36. Shorey S, Pereira TLB, TEO WZ, et al. Navigating nursing curriculum change during COVID-19 pandemic: a systematic review and meta-synthesis. Nurse Educ Pract 2022;65:103483.

37. Leaver CA, Stanley JM, Veenema TG. Impact of the COVID-19 pandemic on the future of nursing education. Academic Medicine 2021. https://doi.org/10.1097/acm.0000000000004528.

38. Omolhoda K, Fahimeh GC, Mahsa K, et al. Clinical nursing education during the COVID-19 pandemic: perspectives of students and clinical educators. BMC Nurs 2022;21:286.

39. Shabsigh R Health. Crisis management in acute care hospitals: lessons learned from COVID-19 and beyond. Springer; 2022. Available at: https://link.springer.com/content/pdf/bfm:978-3-030-95806-0/1?pdf=chapter%20toc.   Accessed August 6, 2023.

40. Wolgast K, Smallheer B. COVID-19 and Pandemic Preparedness: lessons learned and next steps. Nurs Clinic N Amer 2023;58(1). https://doi.org/10.1016/S0029-6465(22)03389-8.

41. Lancet. Pandemic preparedness on all fronts. Lancet Planet Health 2023;7(3). https://doi.org/10.1016/S2542-5196(23)00030-X.

42. Dekker M, van Mansfeld R, Vandenbroucke-Grauls C, et al. Role perception of infection control link nurses; a multicenter qualitative study. J Infect Prev 2022;23(3):93–100.

43. Morley G, Grady C, McCarthy J, et al. COVID-19 ethical challenges for nurses. Hastings Cent Rep 2020;50(3):35–9.

44. American Nurses Association. Crisis standard of care: COVID-19 Pandemic. Retrieve November 1, 2023. Available at: https://www.nursingworld.org/~496044/globalassets/practiceandpolicy/work-environment/health–safety/coronavirus/crisis-standards-of-care.pdf.

45. Kim J, Kim S. Nurses' adaptability in caring for COVID-19 patients: a grounded theory study. Int J Environ Res Publ Health 2021;18(19). https://doi.org/10.3390/ijerph181910141.

46. Labrague L. Psychological resilience, coping behavior and social support among health care workers during the COVID-19 pandemic: a systematic review of quantitative studies. J Nurs Manag 2021;29(7):1893–905.

47. Matusov Y, Matthews A, Rue M, et al. Perceptions of Interdisciplinary collaboration between ICU nurses and resident physicians during the COVID-19 pandemic. J Interprof Educ Pract 2022;27. https://doi.org/10.1016/j.xjep.2022.100501.

48. Arabi Y, Azoulay E, Al-Dorzi H, et al. How the COVID-19 pandemic will change the future of critical care. Intensive Care Med 2021;47(3):282–91.

49. American Nurses Association. COVID-19 Resource Center: Patient Education. Accessed November 1, 2023. Available at: https://www.nursingworld.org/practice-policy/work-environment/health-safety/disaster-preparedness/coronavirus/what-you-need-to-know/clinical-information/patient-education/.

50. Azar K. The evolving role of nurse leadership in the fight for health equity. Nurse Lead 2021;19(6):571–5.

51. Jo S, Kurt S, Bennett J, et al. Nurses' resilience in the face of coronavirus (COVID-19): an international view. Nurs Health Sci 2021;23(3):646–57.

52. Gallo-Cajiao E, Lieberman S, Dolšak N, et al. Global governance for pandemic prevention and the wildlife trade. Lancet Planet Health 2023;7(4):e336–45.

Maslow's Hierarchy of Needs

Achieving Outcomes, Improving Value, and Work Environment - Lessons Learned from the Pandemic

Allison McHugh, DNP, MHCDS, MS, RN, NE-BC[a],*,
Charlene Miller, BSN, RN, CCRN[b],
Christine Stewart, MSN, RN, PHN, CCRN-K, CHTP/I[b]

KEYWORDS

- Nursing practice • Patient outcomes • Work environment • Maslow's hierarchy
- Nursing sensitive outcomes • COVID-19

KEY POINTS

- Describe the significance of a positive work environment on patient and nurse outcomes.
- Describe the impact COVID-19 had on the work environment and routine nursing practice/outcomes in the ICU.
- Describe solutions used to mitigate impacts on nursing practice and how to move forward postpandemic.

Literature has been published on healthy work environments, and its impact on outcomes.[1–5] Yet, in a postpandemic world, we are still trying to improve health care, retention, and employee morale. The impact COVID-19 had on health systems and the work environment is real. Nursing care was impacted by the forces of the pandemic, directly affecting patient outcomes.[6]

This article will provide recommendations on how to move forward in a postpandemic environment to improve nursing practice, our work environment, and nurse-sensitive indicators over the past several years, using Maslow's Hierarchy of Needs as a framework.

MASLOW'S HIERARCHY OF NEEDS

Essentials workers and frontline workers were terms coined during the pandemic of 2020 due to the vital contributions to the crisis of COVID-19. These workers included

[a] Florida State University, Tallahassee, FL, USA; [b] Mercy Medical Center, Redding, CA, USA
* Corresponding author. 98 Varsity Way, Tallahassee, FL 32308.
E-mail address: mchughallison@yahoo.com

Crit Care Nurs Clin N Am 36 (2024) 451–467
https://doi.org/10.1016/j.cnc.2024.02.002
0899-5885/24/© 2024 Elsevier Inc. All rights reserved.

those working in energy, agriculture, grocery stores, transportation, waste, water and teachers, just to name a few[7] Of those, nurses were at the frontline caring for the vulnerable patients suffering from this virus that perplexed the whole country and the proper way to treat it. Debates arose regarding Airborne versus Droplet isolation. Decisions about antivirals; Remdesivir versus Ivermectin, were they safe, were they effective, and were they available? Which population of the ill should receive these drugs? Could they be enrolled in any research studies that were occurring? What drug substitutions were available to combat the drug shortages? How long should a patient be in isolation;10 days or 20 days? Could the deceased donate any organs? It seemed like the public health department, the Food and Drug Administration (FDA), World Health Organization (WHO), and hospital infection control teams were changing practices on a daily basis leading to much confusion and frustration. Nurses had no sense of control.

Some researchers have explored the early impact of the COVID-19 on nursing care delivery broadly in acute care settings ,[8] yet few have concentrated on critical care settings (ICUs).[9]

One Northern California acute care community, level 2 trauma center, like many, has been on a journey to excellence. The hospital has been actively focused on improving outcomes and specifically nurse-sensitive outcomes. Like many other organizations across the United States and beyond, this hospital experienced the significant impact of COVID-19 on its outcomes, both patient and employee. The hospital's ICU is a 29-bed unit with both medical and surgical patients combined, caring for very acute patients in a community whereby the closest Level 1 trauma center is almost 3 hours away. This article will share what was learned from the pandemic related to nursing practice, our work environment, and the progress made postsurge to improve nurse-sensitive patient outcomes over the past several years, focusing on the importance of Maslow's hierarchy of needs.

Maslow's hierarchy of needs is one theory that was written about decades ago, and discusses the importance of essential basic needs being met, for higher level meaning and purpose to be achieved. During the pandemic, several basic needs of nurses were not able to be met; including but not limited to breaks, lunch, and limited resources such as equipment, supplies, and staff. In addition, "feelings of safety were disrupted by personal stressors such as forced societal isolation, disruption in daily routine, unpredictable circumstances, financial uncertainty, and increased needs of adult and child dependents."[10 (p592),11] This hospital, like many, experienced these same struggles: nurse's physical basic needs, safety, and security, a sense of belonging, control, and self-esteem; making it nearly impossible to achieve these most essential needs required to achieve self-actualization[1] In order for nurses to deliver excellent care for patients, their basic needs must be met.

Safety and Security

In 2018, a small ICU in Sweden conducted a yearlong survey of the assessment of the nurses daily reflection of their shift. In this study, they identified 3 common themes of patient safety, workload, and work environment. Data was collected in levels of green, yellow, and red to signify the severity of work conditions, with red being the most severe. Of the levels most reported, workload was consistently at the higher severity levels (yellow and red). Comments that were abstracted from these reflections included not having enough time to complete tasks within a shift and the need to reprioritize during the shift.[12]

This can be said for this Northern California hospital as well. In the beginning of the pandemic, the ICU saw 1 to 2 patients with COVID-19, which allowed for a 1:1 ratio, in order to not expose the other critical patients in the ward. As more cases of COVID-19 occurred, a "zone" approach was adapted to care for these patients. The "hot zone" area was the primary nurse in the patient's room and directly outside the room. Besides caring for the patient, they were responsible for cleaning the patient's room every 4 hours; wiping down the high-touch surfaces and ensuring a clean environment. Charting occurred in the "warm zone," adjacent to the patient's room, with their clean personnel protective equipment (PPE) on, ready to go into a room at any given time. The "warm zone" was also staffed with another nurse or nonlicensed personnel who cleaned the unit, answered call lights, and restocked PPE supplies in the carts. Personnel were available for the hot zone nurse to double bag the garbage from the patient's room. They were also the ones who made sure staff wore their PPE properly and removed it properly. The "cold zone" was a nurse who retrieved supplies from a storage room, pulled meds from the Omnicell for the nurse, monitored the cardiac monitors, and answered the phones. Nurses were also responsible for traffic control, which was one way in and one way out. This experience demonstrated the innovation, efficiency, use of time, and prioritization that were needed to care for such patients during this time. However, nurses' sense of security and ability to complete nursing care were significantly impacted.

During this time, staff were initially instructed to wear simple face masks until test results came back from the laboratory. The looks on the faces of the nurses when they discovered their patient had this new virus that no one knew anything about were heartbreaking. The nurse's eyes were filled with tears, knowing that they had babies at home, who they did not want to expose. Some nurses would sleep away from their families to not put them at risk of being exposed. After further discussion, it was decided to keep the patients in the emergency room until the COVID-19 antigen test resulted, so staff and other patients were not exposed. All of these challenges impacted hospital operations, which created additional emotional and physical stress on staff while trying to keep patients and staff safe. However, efforts were made daily by the leadership to reassure staff and increase communication in real time as much as possible to decrease fears of the unknown.

Self-esteem/Trust and Loss of Trust

Several tough decisions were made that created defeat among many leaders. Vaccinations were a sore spot for many employees because there was so much unknown about the vaccines at the time, and the COVID-19 vaccine was mandatory for employment. Many employees left the organization because of their personal decision not to take part in the vaccination requirements. Employers around the world experienced similar challenges, losing staff, and so forth. However, these issues and many others contributed to staff losing trust in leadership and not feeling cared for. A study by Lord[13] identified that nurses who received a high level of communication regarding COVID-19 were more willing to provide nursing care during the pandemic. This included accurate and timely communication. If their basic safety and security needs were not being met, then how could they deliver good patient care? The impact this loss of trust would have in the long term on the staff and outcomes was significant.

Sense of Belonging

The pandemic gave nurse leaders a whole new level of stressors. They were faced with complex staffing situations as there was a rise in sick calls, ongoing staff shortages, limited bed availability, high patient acuities, and supply shortages, all while trying to support their staff. This led to minimal 1:1 check in's from nursing leadership with staff nurses, which contributed to the staff not feeling supported.

Chen[14] implemented a targeted psychological support program for frontline workers. A chat group was included where one could ask questions and get prompt answers and solutions, a peer communication and sharing network, one-to-one psychological support, targeted themed lectures, daily updates on the latest information about the battle against Covid, and group counseling. Among the participants involved in the program, they felt supported and had a since of belonging to their organization.

Another challenge for staff, was wearing a mask for 2 years. For one full year, staff were required to wear N95's during their 12-h shifts. Thankfully, in March of 2023, the mask mandate was lifted by the public health department, and staff had to get to know their coworkers again as they forgot what they looked like without a mask. Unfortunately, in September of 2023, a rise in COVID-19 cases reoccurred and many frontline workers became sick and missed work. This facility returned to mandatory masking, which was not well received by the staff. However, leadership shared information with staff often, which as described in the literature,[14] relieved some of the anger the staff experienced.

Moral and Ethical Injury

In a national study done by Kissel[15] health care workers working in the ICU reported a rate of anxiety and depression ranging from 19% to 60%, the higher rates were in women. Also reported was a 21.4% rate of burnout among health care workers from May to June 2020. Posttraumatic stress was addressed in this study, in countries such as Canadian, Netherlands, France, and UK PTSD reported at rates of 22%-38%.[15] Many factors contribute to burnout and PTSD.

During the pandemic, caring for families was a great challenge, which also led to significant ethical, moral, and mental stress. Loved ones were restricted from coming to the hospital, and this placed a difficult burden on the health care team. This required the nurse and doctor to call family members daily with updates, sometimes 2 to 3 calls a day. Zoom and Facetime were a learning curve for most. When patients' conditions were eminent, this hospital allowed one family member to be outside the room. This proved to be incredibly stressful for all involved.

In one instance, a patient had been on the rotoprone bed for 14 days and was too unstable to supine. It was absolutely crucial to supine this patient; they needed chest tubes, and the central line and arterial line sites changed. However, in fear that this patient would not tolerate the turn, the wife was brought from out of town to the bedside. The patient survived the supine position during the procedures except for his oxygen saturations, which were maintained in the 60's. After the procedures were complete, the patient was placed into the rotoprone bed, and as the patient was starting to prone, the patient's heart was arrested. The patient was a DNR and was allowed a natural death. The wife, standing on the other side of the glass, was hysterically crying. The nurse quickly removed her PPE to hold the wife in her arms and console her broken heart. The palliative care team was a great resource, as a lot of death was seen day in and day out, which led to significant staff morale and mental distress.

Mental distress was due to a combination of factors such as a loss of safety and security, inadequate staffing levels, and no time to care for oneself. As described here and as many authors describe, the importance of achieving Maslow's hierarchy of needs is crucial to achieving self-actualization, which allows one to implement ideas, affirm one's role, rise to the moment, and fulfill professional potential.[10] If leaders want to learn one thing about the pandemic, meeting the nurses' most basic needs is always a wonderful place to start. Making this a priority is something that should be at the core of our profession. We care for other people for a living, which is why it is important that nurses in turn are cared for. Additional strategies that have been shown to improve nurse's well-being include taking time to reflect daily on the activities of the shift and to participate in psychological support groups.[14]

HEALTHY WORK ENVIRONMENT

A healthy work environment is essential for the success and desirable outcomes of any organization. However, when the employees basic needs are not met, this makes it more difficult to promote a healthy work environment. (Raso, 2022), making it even more challenging to achieve successful outcomes, including patient satisfaction, quality, and employee satisfaction. If our nurses' work environment and basic needs are not met, patient care will suffer, therefore, we must address and nurture them and their environment.[16]

In an article by Selanders,[16] Nightingale 's theory of environmental adaptation discussed the significant impact the physical environment has on patient outcomes. Florence Nightingale, in her famous notes on nursing (1860), states, "if a patient is cold, if a patient is feverish, if a patient is faint, if he is sick after taking food, if he has a bed sore, it is generally the fault not of the disease, but of the nursing"[16 (p6)] To some, this statement might feel harsh, but what it says to other professions, is our work *matters*. The nurses' work brings value and is essential to improving patient outcomes. The implication is clear, the nurse is responsible for maintaining the environment in such a manner as to maintain the health of the patient.

A healthy work environment has been described by the American Association of Critical-Care Nursing (AACN) and others as comprising skilled communication, true collaboration, effective decision-making, appropriate staffing, meaningful recognition, and authentic leadership.[17] These standards must be in place to create and ensure a healthy work environment and provide an evidence-based framework for any organization committed to excellence and improving patient outcomes.[18] The second edition of these standards was published in 2016, to incorporate additional evidence to support the relationship between a healthy work environment and improved outcomes for patients and nurses.[17 (p168)].

IMPLICIT RATIONING/MISSED CARE/OMITTED CARE/DIMINISHED NURSING CARE

During COVID-19, not only was the work environment significantly impacted, but the conditions nurses and other care givers worked in created an environment whereby necessary care interventions were not able to be provided. Otherwise stated, care was often missed or omitted because implicit rationing was occurring. Implicit rationing, however, has been described in the literature, long before COVID-19.[19–21] Research has demonstrated the significance of the presence of implicit rationing and poor patient outcomes, as well as the inverse relationship between healthy work environments and the presence of implicit rationing[22] As previously mentioned, the pandemic created many opportunities for the work environment to remain "unhealthy," this included staffing, collaboration, decision making, and recognition.

McHugh[23] implemented an evidenced-based practice project, looking at the work environment and its impact on implicit rationing, during the pandemic. A survey was conducted at this hospital with IRB approval, using the AACN Healthy Work Environment Assessment Tool.

(HWEAT)[24] and the perceived implicit the rationing of nursing care assessment (PIRNCA).[25] Several of the standards present in a healthy work environment were not perceived by nurses as being met in many of the units, such as adequate staffing, meaningful recognition, and collaboration. The healthy work environment subscales (**Table 1**) display each unit's scores using the HWEAT. As seen in **Table 1**, the nurses in the ICU specifically reported all areas of the work environment as "not healthy."

This project also surveyed nurses in the adult acute care and critical care units using the PIRNCA to assess for the presence of implicit rationing. The PIRNCA is a tool that asks nurses to report how often, in the last 7 shifts, they were able to complete specific nursing interventions. Based on the nurses report, a percentage is calculated, demonstrating the presence of implicit rationing by unit.[25] The results of this project demonstrated the existence of an inverse relationship, between work environment and implicit rationing. **Table 2** demonstrates how often specific nursing care activities were not able to be completed by each unit including; basic needs with physical care such as turning, mobility, and skin care. This data aligns with the qualitative reports of the nurses' lived experiences in the ICU. Results of this survey were shared with the nurse managers and leaders in April 2022, and an educational intervention was implemented to increase the awareness and importance of healthy work environments as it applies to implicit rationing.

NURSE-SENSITIVE OUTCOMES, STANDARDS OF CARE AND THE IMPACT OF COVID-19 ON NURSING PRACTICE

Standards of care were impacted during the pandemic due to significant disruptions in the nurse's workflow and practice. Authors such as Grimley,[6] and Patel,[26] discuss this impact on practice in hospitals across the United States and beyond. Some of these included but were not limited to; assessing patients from windows versus having face-to-face contact, being in fear of infecting oneself, limiting the adherence to best practices and rigor in the interventions of care that were to be performed. In the early phases of the pandemic, in an effort to reduce exposure to employees, this facility temporarily paused the practice of direct observations, looking at central line care and Foley catheter care. Later, it was discovered that there was an increase in hospital-acquired infections. The significance of these direct observations in practice was critical.

Because improving value not only improves quality, it does so while also assuming a decrease in cost. Therefore, it is important to describe the cost of hospital-acquired conditions. The Agency for Healthcare Research and Quality (AHRQ)[27] reports the average cost of hospital-acquired conditions include.

- Catheter-associated Urinary Tract Infections (CAUTI)- $13,793 ($5019–$22,568)
- Central- Line-Associated Blood Stream Infections (CLABSI)- $48,108 ($27,232–$68,983)
- Hospital-Acquired Pressure Injuries (HAPIs)- $14,506 (-$14,506–$41,326)

Hospitals across the country receive financial reimbursement, which is heavily reliant on these outcomes. Therefore, it is critical for nurses to understand the value their work has on these outcomes from both a quality and safety perspective and financial perspective. The practice of nursing improves outcomes, which decreases hospital-acquired conditions, promoting significant value to the health care system.

Nurses as stewards of the health care system need to understand the significance of their work and the impact it has on quality and cost. A nurse's care and interventions can prevent hospital-acquired conditions, reduce unnecessary harm to patients, and decrease hospital costs. This can save a hospital hundreds of thousands of dollars, which could be used on other expenses, such as investing in new equipment for care delivery and innovation.

Table 1
Unit healthy work environment subscales

Unit	Nurses	Skilled Communication	Collaboration	Decision- Making	Staffing	Meaningful Recognition	Authentic Leadership
Total N	70	3.20	2.91	3.28	2.83	2.96	3.32
Unit I	8	3.63	3.50	3.88	3.48	3.75	3.79
Unit 2	14	3.76	3.43	3.64	3.43	3.38	3.71
Unit 3	17	3.08	2.75	3.33	2.82	2.82	3.45
Unit 4	2	2.83	2.83	3.17	3.00	2.33	3.50
Unit 5	19	2.72	2.40	2.81	2.02	2.40	2.77
Unit 6	1	2.00	2.0	1.67	2.00	2.33	2.33
Unit 7	2	3.83	3.67	4.17	4.00	3.17	3.83
Unit 8	7	3.29	2.95	3.00	2.95	3.24	3.10

Note. Adapted from[23] (p68)

Table 2
Unit percentage of implicit rationing (IR)

Item#	Nursing Care Activity	%IR all Units	Unit 1	Unit 2	Unit 3	Unit 4	Unit 5	Unit 6	Unit 7	Unit 8
Assist with physical care		86.89								
6	Timely assist with bowel/bladder	85.7	62.5	76.9	93.8	100	85.7	100	100	100
1	Routine hygiene	90.5	87.5	76.9	100	100	85.7	100	100	100
5	Mobility or changing position	88.9	75	76.9	93.8	100	92.9	100	100	100
4	Ambulate with assistance	92	87.5	92.3	100	100	78.6	100	100	100
3	Changing soiled linen	84	87.5	53.8	93.8	100	85.7	100	100	100
2	Routine skin care	88.9	87.5	84.6	93.8	100	78.6	100	100	100
7	Assist with po intake fluid/food	84.1	75	76.9	81.3	100	85.7	100	100	100
8	Promoting physical comfort	81	62.5	61.5	87.5	100	85.7	100	100	71.4
Monitoring safety support		69.46								
18	Monitoring physiologic status	58.7	62.5	61.5	62.5	100	28.6	100	50	85.7
19	Monitoring behavior	64.5	62.5	61.5	60	100	57	100	50	100
17	Emotional or psychological support	82.3	42.9	69.2	93.8	100	85.7	100	50	85.7
13	Compliance with safe patient handling	76.2	50	69.2	68.8	100	92.9	0	50	57.1
16	Prep for test, treatment	71.4	50	53.8	81.3	100	71.4	100	100	100
20	Monitoring physical safety	64.5	50	69.2	60	100	50	0	50	100
15	Teaching for patient and family safety	76.2	75	46.2	87.5	100	78.6	100	100	85.7
21	Follow up on patient status change	61.9	50	46.2	62.5	100	64.3	100	100	100
Documentation supervision		75.65								
30	Documentation of all nursing care	84.1	75	69.2	81.2	100	100	100	100	85.7
31	Evaluation of plan of care	69.8	62.5	38.5	75	100	78.6	100	100	85.7
29	Documentation of assessments	71.4	75	61.5	62.5	100	78.6	100	100	85.7

Note. *Adapted from*[23] (pp69-70)

Central Line-associated Blood Stream Infections

During the pandemic, specifically at its peak, (spring 2020), central line use was increased due to the instability of the patients. After several increased cases of central line infections, a deeper dive was taken by leadership in the ICU and this hospital, including administration and the quality department, to understand the causes specific to the pandemic. Nursing and physician practices were modified from evidenced-based practice guidelines due to the acuity and changing work environment as noted later in discussion.

Central lines were placed for emergent vasopressors and sedation. During multidisciplinary rounds there was disagreement among physicians who preferred to keep central lines in the patient longer in case the patient declined. Proning these patients was often a requirement due to their acuity. This made access to the central line site difficult to access, therefore sites were not accurately assessed, and it was difficult to effectively care for these lines. This included 2% chlorhexidine gluconate (CHG) baths not being completed on a daily basis. Patients requiring proning therapy had an increase in secretions which often flowed into the central line site. The increase in moisture leads to central line dressings becoming loose leading to more exposure of bacteria.

Because staff had to weigh the risks of infecting themselves, and keeping the patients safe, innovation was implemented to limit the frequent exposure in the rooms. For all these reasons, this created a barrier to frequent assessments of the lines. Central line infection rates increased during the pandemic, 2020 to 2021 due to the many disruptions in the work environment and nursing practice setting. However, in 2022, these decreased, and currently, the hospital's ICU has gone well over a year, since the last CLABSI, which has been celebrated and acknowledged.

Fakih[28] conducted a study that demonstrated the difference in CLABSI rates "compared to the period before the COVID-19 pandemic, and CLABSI rates increased by 51.0% during the pandemic period from 0.56 to 0.85 per 1000 line days ($P < .001$) and by 62.9% from 1.00 to 1.64 per 10,000 patient days ($P < .001$)". This study also stated that "hospitals with monthly COVID-19 patients representing greater than 10% of admissions had a National Health Safety Network (NHSN) device standardized infection ratio for CLABSI that was 2.38 times higher than hospitals with less than 5% prevalence during the pandemic period ($P=.004$)."[28] What this reinforces is the significant importance of hardwiring processes and providing regular feedback on performance, to maintain a safe environment.[28]

Catheter-associated Urinary Tract Infections

Keeping track of strict intake and output (I&O's) was an important intervention for these critically ill patients. This led to an increased use of Foley catheters. This facility uses an evidenced-based nurse-driven protocol, giving the bedside nurse autonomy to discontinue a Foley catheter if the patient no longer meets criteria. During the pandemic, nursing tended to keep Foleys in longer, even if they necessarily did not meet criteria. This allowed staff to monitor I&Os from the door rather than increasing their exposure. The proning position posed difficulty not just on central lines but on Foley catheters as well, making it problematic to perform peri care appropriately. Another problem nurses encountered was the use of securement devices for the Foley catheters. If properly placed and when a patient was proned, it led to a risk of device-related pressure injury. However, when the catheters were not secured, this could lead to the catheter getting pulled on frequently, which could have contributed to an increase in CAUTIs. An academic medical center in the Midwest who cared for more than 6000 patients with COVID-19 developed a CAUTI committee and new standards of care for their COVID population. One of the standards was to make sure that drainage bags were emptied prior to any repositioning. This prevented any backflow of urine into the bladder. They also made it a new standard to remove the securement device from the anterior thigh and replace it on the posterior thigh after the patient was placed in the prone position. All patients received a full-body CHG bath treatment while in the supine position along with catheter care.[29]

This facility developed a "Ticket to Test" for urinalysis with reflex to culture testing. This gave staff guidance on criteria for indications to send a urinalysis and criteria that do meet indications, such as sending a sample on a patient who is experiencing dysuria, urgency, or frequency within 48 hours after having an indwelling catheter removed. These guidelines have decreased unnecessary treatment for patients. In 2020 to 2021, due to COVID-19 and the disruptions in nursing practice routines, CAUTI rates increased. However, the rate has significantly decreased since these best practices have returned. This hospital's ICU has gone well over a year with no CAUTI.

Hospital-acquired pressure injuries

Proning was another challenge that most hospitals around the globe faced during the pandemic. The prone position is when a patient is turned face down in the bed, which helps improve lung function. Typically, rotoprone beds are a specialty bed used in caring for patients who need to be proned. However, as COVID-19 numbers were rising throughout this state, rotoprone beds were extremely limited. Some patients were put on a waiting list for this specialty bed. This led to staff having to manually prone patients. This skill took specific training for the nurses. To properly and safely prone a ventilated patient, six health care workers and a respiratory therapist were necessary. As one could imagine, this was a difficult feat. A turn team was trialed using resources throughout the hospital. Daily in the leadership safety meeting, it was announced how many resources were needed that day to assist with proning. Senior leadership and administration could be found in the ICU from time to time to help prone patients. However, there were times when staffing was extremely limited, and staff would prone patients with the minimum resources.

Staff were tired, exhausted, beyond what we had ever seen. Defeated. Due to the nature of their acuity, some of these patients had extensive periods of proning, up to 16 hours at a time. Many of these patients were hemodynamically unstable, requiring vasopressors. These patients were difficult to ventilate at times, which led to decreased perfusion to the skin, therefore increasing their risk for pressure injuries.

It was difficult to find the best way to prevent HAPIs on the face area, particularly the lips, cheeks, and nose, while these patients were prone. Different facial pillows were trialed, strategic placement of preventive dressings with premade cut outs were made available for easier use, education on the "swimmer position," and controversy on the safety of using tape on endotracheal tubes were areas of focus. Despite the efforts of the staff, many of these patients suffered a HAPI to the face due to long prone times, pressor requirements, and tissue death.

Pressure injuries specific to the coccyx also increased during COVID, due to the inability to effectively turn and offload patients, and the limited resources resulting from the nationwide strain of the pandemic. To meet the needs of increasing patients with COVID-19 requiring isolation, hospital rooms were converted into negative pressure rooms, causing the rooms to be very warm, creating moist environments for patients' skin. Staff were extremely discouraged by these outcomes. Some staff were disappointed in their peers, others felt some staff just stopped caring, others felt it was the increased number of travelers, some just felt there was no purpose; and others did what they could to just get through the shift because of pure exhaustion and burnout along with limited staff. Ultimately these events may have been prevented by effective offloading with more available resources to properly turn patients. As many hospitals experienced during COVID-19 2020 to 2021, the pressure injury rates increased due to the factors described; however, the rates have decreased over time.

MOVING FORWARD

Postpandemic, *direct observations* have returned, concentrating on evidence-based practice. Things addressed in these observations are central line dressing integrity, line care, and site condition. A staff member of the ICU has been recruited to be our central line champion. This staff member comes in once a week (same day each week), changes all central line dressings, and audits the lines and dressings. This allows for peer-to-peer feedback on any practice deficiencies. Foley catheters are observed for positioning and preventing dependent lopes, use of stat lock, and pericare documentation as well.

Postpandemic this hospital has developed a committee that meets once a week and discusses that week's falls, skin issues, and safe patient handling. This allows leaders to group together and discuss diverse ways to prevent harm to the patients.

As discussed, the work environment significantly contributes to patient outcomes and the conditions that allow nurses to deliver the care necessary for safe, quality care. Articles such as Patel,[25] Weiner-Lastinger,[30] Grimley,[6] and Fakih,[28] demonstrate that hospitals across the country and globe were impacted by the pandemic. What this also demonstrates is the significant importance of the work of the nurse. Nursing care prevents harm. Implicit rationing occurred during the pandemic at rates that were not scientifically captured but are worth studying in the future in further detail. The conditions in work environments across the country produced the "perfect storm" for nurses to be placed in positions whereby they had to ration care given the limited resources available during the pandemic. Since literature supports the association between work environment and implicit rationing,[22] it is critical for leaders and nurses to be educated on the importance of understanding what is contributing to changes in patient outcomes. Then closely examine the environment to understand factors that could be preventing the care being provided, that is, implicit rationing. If the environment creates conditions such that a nurse must choose which care to provide and what not to provide, this is a problem that must be addressed. It is important to inform both nurse leaders and nurses about implicit rationing and its impact on patient outcomes.

RECOMMENDATIONS
How We lead: The Nurse Leaders Role in Improving the Work Environment and Basic Needs

Although COVID-19 dramatically changed health care in many ways, including our health care environment, we can no longer continue to use that as a reason to not make improvements or to not use our experiences from COVID- 19 to become better and more prepared for the future. Nurses learned to innovate, to think out of the box, to identify what was needed and what was not, along with thinking about new care delivery models. So, how do we move forward and emerge from the pandemic? We need to take what we learned and apply it to our practice, now.

Starting with the role of the nurse leader in committing to understanding the work environment and the conditions nurses are working in, the presence of implicit rationing, along with implementing strategies to support the emotional health of the workforce. Leaders must commit to understanding Maslow's hierarchy of needs and so do nurses.

We learned from the literature and direct reports, that nurses did not feel heard, communicated to, valued, or recognized, and they did not feel they were able to play a role in decision making regarding their practice, and certainly nurses did not feel like they were part of a team that was collaborative. It has also been described and demonstrated in the literature, that the nurses work impacts outcomes and if the nurse and their environment is not cared for, their care will negatively impact patient outcomes. If the literature supports the importance of collaboration, communication, shared decision making among other things such as recognition, then why was this so difficult?

What do nurses want from leaders ?

- Leaders who are present, leaders who listen, take their opinion and ideas into consideration
- Leaders who allow innovation but also hold staff accountable to standards of practice
- Leaders who are dedicated to improving the work environment
- Leaders they can trust, who care about them, appreciate them, and celebrate them as people, those who have a genuine sense of care for their well-being as evidenced by role modeling
- Leaders who instill a sense of authenticity, hope, inspiration, joy, calmness, and support

This article supports the need for nursing and nurse leaders to focus on further understanding what is happening in their work environment, focusing on the basic needs of the staff, infrastructure, resources, practices, and how this is impacting patient outcomes. It is important for nurses to also understand the concept of implicit rationing and to be empowered to speak up about what they need to influence their ability to practice and deliver the evidenced-based care that is required for desired outcomes. The literature has demonstrated repeatedly the significance the work of a nurse has on patient outcomes and our results also demonstrate the impact of outcomes when the environment is not conducive to this care delivery. COVID-19 highlighted this across the country, but what has been learned from this experience? It is our hope that from this tragedy, nursing practice will continue to improve, leaders and nurses will regain trust and pride in the profession, and patient outcomes will outperform any benchmark. It will also be important for future leaders to conduct additional observational studies to demonstrate the value that the work of the nurse brings to patient outcomes, including understanding implicit rationing in the work environment.

How We Care for Self and One Another

In 2017, the Institute for Health Care improvement released an article "Improving Joy in the workplace."[31] This was pre-COVID-19, and the framework was simple. Ask your employees what is getting in the way of JOY. What do they need to be able to have more JOY at work? We need leaders and organizations that demonstrate a true commitment to improving JOY in the workplace every day. Organizations such as the American Organization for Nurse Leaders (AONL), the American Nurses Association (ANA), and Association of Leadership Science in Nursing (ALSN) support the ongoing work of improving the work environment. What needs continued commitment by nurse leaders and nurses are the ability to engage, empower, and be involved in shared decision making related to nursing practice, work environment redesign, and involvement in health care policy changes. Some of these should include funding for specialty hospitals for mental health, increasing alternatives for access to care, and consistent incentives from insurance companies to drive down costs and increase quality.

It is important to reflect on the high rate of depression and burn out in nurses and nurse leaders *prior* to COVID-19, and to understand how these mental health conditions and other factors, such as low morale, poor staffing, implicit rationing, and unhealthy work environments exacerbated traumatic emotional responses in nursing staff. In a 2022 article, "Beyond Burnout and Resilience the Disillusionment Phase of COVID-19," Gee[32] discusses the emotional toll of compassion fatigue, secondary trauma, moral distress, cumulative grief, burnout, and PTSD on nurses. Prior to the pandemic, nurses were known to have a higher rate of burnout and depression than other professions. COVID-19 exacerbated these conditions, with one study revealing that many nurses were planning to decrease their work hours, and up to 40% were planning to leave nursing altogether within 2 years.[32]

Understanding this mental health crisis in the workforce and taking action to facilitate education on proven resilience skills such as mindfulness and gratitude practices, is an important part of moving forward to create a stronger, healthier work environment by creating stronger, healthier nurses. It is incumbent on nursing leadership to set the example by demonstrating self-care practices and by recognizing and communicating the need for self-care by nurses. The Greater Good Science Center at UC Berkeley[33] noted that simple steps such as a nurse writing down something they are grateful for twice per week, showed a 28% decrease in perceived stress, and a 16% decrease in depression. Using gratitude practices during daily shift huddles, and/or saying "thank you" to employees can increase feelings of trust and increase productivity by as much as 50%.[33] These shared practices have the added advantage of team building and can be instrumental in driving culture change toward a healthy work environment.

Not only do we have to find ways to care for ourselves and each other, but a recommended emphasis would also include training for the succession planning of both leaders and bedside nurses. Other strategies such as learning techniques that support mindfulness and self-care "resilience small groups," like the Center for Mind Body Medicine (CMBM)[34] can be instrumental in teaching leaders and nurses the best ways to maintain resilience and ways to be ready for any tragedy.

How We Care for Our Patients

As mentioned previously, it has been shown that the nurses reflect daily on their shift is important to them. In this hospital, during daily huddles, staff are given time to "shout out" and recognize their colleagues. Continuous work is underway focusing on the culture in the ICU, using self-assessment tools to reflect on one's own behavior, and using skills such as HRO (high-reliability organization) in the nurses' day-to-day practices. As leaders, the goal is to create an environment that is a safe place to speak up and share concerns as appropriate. This ICU also started a "good catch" program whereby staff and leaders can recommend a colleague to keep patient safety at the fore front. As described in the literature, positive reinforcement and recognition contribute to a healthy work environment, which produce the conditions for nurses to thrive in and therefore provide excellent care and outcomes.

Along with the continuation of the direct observations of Healthcare Associated Infection (HAI) prevention, staff are educated on new developments in evidenced-based practice and the development or changes to protocols and procedures. Staff have access to applications that allow them admittance to specific policies regarding nursing practice within the organization. Within these there are many publications on evidence-based practice available to staff. Annual employee survey results are shared with the staff, and collaborative discussions are held regarding the unfavorable results. Staff assist in developing action plans toward improvements. Town hall meetings have returned postpandemic to ensure that staff members have knowledge of the direction the organization is going and gain answers to any questions they may have. These strategies contribute to improving collaboration, communication, and shared decision making, all factors that support a healthy work environment.

Focusing on an ICU that provides patient-family-centered care has been a priority for this facility. Moving forward, we learned that patient-family-centered care is important even in the event of COVID-19. At this facility, a designated family member is allowed at the bedside with the understanding that it is recommended to limit their exposure and are required to wear PPE in the room. Family members are also encouraged to be present for multidisciplinary rounds, which helps with communication and understanding.

Recently, this facility had an ICU reunion whereby patients who survived COVID-19 returned to the hospital to tell their story. This allowed staff to see the wonderful work they are doing, and it is a terrific way for staff to fill their cup hearing from patients they cared for and the impact they made on their care. In this reunion, it was discovered that 2 strangers, family members of the patients, connected and were each other's support network. These patients volunteer their time and function as a support person for others in need. The unit has also developed an ICU diary to assist the families in recalling the confusing time while in the hospital, and it has been shown to help with Postintensive care syndrome (PICS), which helps the patient recall the lost time while they were in the hospital.

FUTURE RESEARCH CONSIDERATIONS

This article provides insight regarding the importance of the work of the nurse on patient outcomes. Specifically, what was learned from the pandemic related to nursing practice and the impact the work environment has on patient and nursing outcomes. Future research should be considered in the areas of further exploring implicit rationing and the work environment, in critical care and acute care, using reliable, valid tools such as the PIRNCA, and through the use of observational studies.

SUMMARY

The pandemic highlighted the importance of a healthy work environment for patient outcomes. It also demonstrated the significance of the presence of Maslow's hierarchy of needs for nurses to achieve self-actualization and be able to deliver their best selves. The work of nursing matters, and we must continue to focus on the work environment. Ulrich,[17] described that 71% of nurses and nurse leaders reported either "just beginning" or "not at all" related to implementing the AACN healthy work environment standards. One of the reasons these standards were not implemented was that "other health care executives were not familiar with healthy work environments."[17] This is our time to act, communicate, collaborate, and change the work environment together, with all our colleagues in the health care profession, improving outcomes for patients, health care professionals, and communities.

Although nursing practice is the sole focus of this article, it cannot go unnoticed that other factors contribute to the conditions of the work environment that must be fixed, including but not limited to, the many operational inefficiencies and their cost. The root cause of these problems and the patient and employee outcomes that have been impacted the most due to the impacts of COVID-19, must be understood.

Additional priorities should also include developing health policies to support reimbursements that can reflect care delivery. Focusing on partnerships with insurance companies that help health care organizations achieve health promotion and design programs with incentives. Such as those that stimulate growth, allow health care professionals to thrive, innovate, and reduce harm, while promoting quality at the lowest cost.

People should always be first. If we take care of our people, they will take care of our patients and the outcomes will follow, clinically, operationally, and in the end financially. Hospitals will continue to struggle financially if they do not prioritize retention, resilience, engagement, work environment, and leadership. This is our time to shine, collaborate, communicate, engage, innovate, inspire, and deliver outcomes.

CLINICS CARE POINTS

- Work environment significantly impacts patient outcomes and implicit rationing
- Nursing practice significantly impacts patient outcomes
- The importance of Maslow's hierarchy of needs on nursing practice

DISCLOSURE

The authors have nothing to disclose.

REFERENCES

1. Faerber A, Andrews A, Lobb A, et al. A new model of online health care delivery science education for mid-career health care professionals. Healthc (Amst) 2019; 7(4). S2213-0764(17)30247-6.
2. Berwick DM, Nolan TW, Whittington J. The triple aim: care, health, and cost. Health Aff 2008;27(3):759–69.
3. Wei H, Sewell KA, Woody G, et al. The state of the science of nurse work environments in the United States: a systematic review. Int J Nurs Sci 2018;5(3):287–300.
4. Mihdawi M, Al-Amer R, Darwish R, et al. The influence of nursing work environment on patient safety. Workplace Health & Saf 2020;68(8):384–90.
5. Copanitsanou P, Fotos N, Brokalaki H. Effects of work environment on patient and nurse outcomes. Br J Nurs 2017;26(3):172–6.
6. Grimley KA, Gruebling N, Kurani A, et al. Nurse sensitive indicators and how COVID-19 influenced practice change. Nurse Lead 2021;19(4):371–7.
7. COVID-19: essential workers in the states. 2023. Available at: https://www.ncsl.org/labor-and-employment/Covid-19-essential-workers-in-the-states.
8. Schroeder K, Norful AA, Travers J, et al. Nursing perspectives on care delivery during the early stages of the Covid-19 pandemic: a qualitative study. Int J Nurs Stud Adv 2020;2:100006.
9. Bethel C, Rainbow JG, Johnson K. A qualitative descriptive study of the COVID-19 pandemic: impacts on nursing care delivery in the critical care work system. Appl Ergon 2022;102:103712.
10. Hayre-Kwan S, Quinn B, Chu T, et al. Nursing and Maslow's hierarchy: a health care pyramid approach to safety and security during a global pandemic. Nurse Lead 2021;19(6):590–5.

11. Raso R. Rebuilding our workforce: revisiting Maslow's hierarchy. Nurs Manag 2022;53(8):5.

12. Larsson IM, Aronsson A, Norén K, et al. Healthcare workers' structured daily reflection on patient safety, workload and work environment in intensive care. A descriptive retrospective study. Intensive Crit Care Nurs 2022;68:103122.

13. Lord H, Loveday C, Moxham L, et al. Effective communication is key to intensive care nurses' willingness to provide nursing care amidst the COVID-19 pandemic. Intensive Crit Care Nurs 2021;62:102946.

14. Chen SH, Liu JE, Bai XY, et al. Providing targeted psychological support to front-line nurses involved in the management of COVID-19: an action research. J Nurs Manag 2021;29(5):1169–79.

15. Kissel KA, Filipek C, Jenkins J. Impact of the COVID-19 pandemic on nurses working in intensive care units: a scoping review. Crit Care Nurse 2023;43(2):55–63.

16. Selanders LC. The power of environmental adaptation: florence Nightingale's original theory for nursing practice. J Holist Nurs 2010;28(1):81–8.

17. Ulrich B, Barden C, Cassidy L, et al. Critical care nurse work environments 2018: findings and implications. Crit Care Nurse 2019;39(2):67–84.

18. Available at:AACN standards for establishing and sustaining healthy work environments. A journey to excellence. 2nd edition. American Association of Critical Care Nurses; 2016 www.aacn.org.

19. Jones TL, Hamilton P, Murry N. Unfinished nursing care, missed care, and implicitly rationed care: state of the science review. Int J Nurs Stud 2015;52(6):1121–37.

20. Dhaini SR, Simon M, Ausserhofer D, et al. Trends and variability of implicit rationing of care across time and shifts in an acute care hospital: a longitudinal study. J Nurs Manag 2020;28(8):1861–72.

21. Zúñiga F, Ausserhofer D, Hamers JP, et al. The relationship of staffing and work environment with implicit rationing of nursing care in Swiss nursing homes–A cross-sectional study. Int J Nurs Stud 2015;52(9):1463–74.

22. Zhao Y, Ma D, Wan Z, et al. Associations between work environment and implicit rationing of nursing care: a systematic review. J Nurs Manag 2020;28(8):1841–50.

23. McHugh A. The Nursing Leader's Role in Decreasing Implicit Rationing by Improving the Nursing Work Environment. University Las Vegas Nevada, DNP Publication as Degree Project with UNLV; 2022.

24. American Association of Critical Care Nurses. AACN healthy work environment assessment tool. American Association of Critical Care Nurses website. Available at: https://www.aacn.org/nursing-excellence/healthy-work-environments/aacn-healthy-work-environment-assessment-tool.

25. Jones TL. Validation of the perceived implicit rationing of nursing care (PIRNCA) instrument. Nurs Forum 2014;49(2):77–87.

26. Patel PR, Weiner-Lastinger LM, Dudeck MA, et al. Impact of COVID-19 pandemic on central-line-associated bloodstream infections during the early months of 2020, National Healthcare Safety Network. Infect Control Hosp Epidemiol 2022; 43(6):790–3.

27. Estimating the additional hospital inpatient cost and mortality associated with selected hospital-acquired conditions. Rockville, MD: Agency for Healthcare Research and Quality; 2017. Available at: https://www.ahrq.gov/hai/pfp/haccost2017.html.

28. Fakih MG, Bufalino A, Sturm L, et al. Coronavirus disease 2019 (COVID-19) pandemic, central-line-associated bloodstream infection (CLABSI), and catheter-associated urinary tract infection (CAUTI): the urgent need to refocus on hardwiring prevention efforts. Infect Control Hosp Epidemiol 2022;43(1):26–31.

29. Stifter J, Sermersheim E, Ellsworth M, et al. COVID-19 and nurse-sensitive indicators: using performance improvement teams to address quality indicators during a pandemic. J Nurs Care Qual 2021;36(1):1–6.
30. Weiner-Lastinger LM, Pattabiraman V, Konnor RY, et al. The impact of coronavirus disease 2019 (COVID-19) on healthcare-associated infections in 2020: a summary of data reported to the National Healthcare Safety Network [published correction appears in Infect Control Hosp Epidemiol. 2022 Jan;43(1):137]. Infect Control Hosp Epidemiol 2022;43(1):12–25.
31. Perlo J, Balik B, Swensen S, et al. IHI Framework for improving Joy in work;2017; IHI White Paper. Cambridge, Massachusetts: Institute for Healthcare Improvement. Available at: https://www.ncha.org/wp-content/uploads/2018/06/IHIWhite Paper_FrameworkForImprovingJoyInWork.pdf
32. Gee PM, Weston MJ, Harshman T, et al. Beyond burnout and resilience: the disillusionment phase of COVID-19. AACN Adv Crit Care 2022;33(2):134–42.
33. Greater good science center. Gratitude practice for nurses: a toolkit for well-being. 2021. Available at: https://ggsc.berkeley.edu/images/uploads/Gratitude_Nurses_Toolkit.pdf.
34. The center for Mind- body medicine. Available at: https://cmbm.org/self-care-resources.

Moving?

Make sure your subscription moves with you!

To notify us of your new address, find your **Clinics Account Number** (located on your mailing label above your name), and contact customer service at:

Email: journalscustomerservice-usa@elsevier.com

800-654-2452 (subscribers in the U.S. & Canada)
314-447-8871 (subscribers outside of the U.S. & Canada)

Fax number: 314-447-8029

Elsevier Health Sciences Division
Subscription Customer Service
3251 Riverport Lane
Maryland Heights, MO 63043

*To ensure uninterrupted delivery of your subscription, please notify us at least 4 weeks in advance of move.

Printed and bound by CPI Group (UK) Ltd, Croydon, CR0 4YY

08/05/2025

01864724-0010